Mayo Clinic on
High Blood Pressure

About the editor-in-chief

Dr. Sheldon G. Sheps is an emeritus professor of medicine at Mayo Medical School. He was a member of Mayo Clinic's cardiovascular diseases consulting staff for 37 years before retiring from clinical practice in 1997. From 1990 to 1996 he was chair of Mayo Clinic's Division of Hypertension and Internal Medicine.

Dr. Sheps has served on many national committees devoted to the treatment and prevention of high blood pressure and other vascular diseases. He has edited several textbooks and authored numerous scientific articles. From 1996 to 1997, Dr. Sheps chaired the group that developed the Sixth Report of the Joint National Committee on the Prevention, Detection, Evaluation and Treatment of High Blood Pressure. The report is an educational tool for primary care providers sponsored by the National Heart, Lung, and Blood Institute, a division of the National Institutes of Health.

For his many contributions toward improving high blood pressure education and awareness, in 1997 Dr. Sheps received the Individual Achievement Award from the National High Blood Pressure Education Program, part of the National Heart, Lung, and Blood Institute.

Mayo Clinic on High Blood Pressure

Sheldon G. Sheps, M.D.
Editor-in-Chief

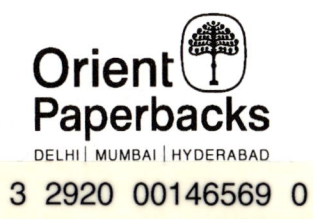

Mayo Clinic on High Blood Pressure provides reliable, practical, easy-to-understand information on preventing and managing high blood pressure. Much of the information comes directly from the experience of Mayo Clinic physicians, nurses, registered dietitians, health educators and other health care professionals. This book supplements the advice of your personal physician, whom you should consult for individual medical problems. Mayo Clinic on High Blood Pressure does not endorse any company or product. Mayo and Mayo Clinic are marks of Mayo Foundation for Medical Education and Research.

All rights reserved. No part of this publication may be reproduced or transmitted in any form or by any means, electronic or mechanical, including photocopying and recording, or introduced into any information storage and retrieval system without the written permission of the copyright owner and the publisher of this book. Brief quotations may be used in reviews prepared for inclusion in a magazine, newspaper, or broadcast. For further information, please contact Orient Paperbacks, Madarsa Road, Kashmere Gate, Delhi-110 006. Tel: (011) 2386 2201, 2386 2267 Fax: (011) 2386 2935

Menu analysis was done by Mayo Clinic registered dietitians using nutritionist IV software by N-Squared.

www.orientpaperbacks.com

ISBN 81-222-0282-9

1st Published 2001
4th Printing 2005

Mayo Clinic on High Blood Pressure

© 1999 Mayo Foundation for Medical
Education and Research

Published in arrangement with
Mayo Foundation for Medical
Education and Research, USA

The logo and trademark 'Good Health First' are owned by
Orient Paperbacks, a division of Vision Books Pvt. Ltd.

Published by
Orient Paperbacks
(A division of Vision Books Pvt. Ltd.)
Madarsa Road, Kashmere Gate, Delhi-110 006

Printed at
Ravindra Printing Press, Delhi-110 006

About High Blood Pressure

One in four adults in the United States has high blood pressure. You or a family member may be one of them.

High blood pressure is a deceptive illness because it causes few, if any, symptoms. That's why many people, perhaps even you, don't view it as a life-threatening condition. Nothing could be further from the truth. High blood pressure is a leading cause of stroke, heart attack, heart failure, kidney failure and premature death. If you don't take it seriously, it can shorten your life by 10 to 20 years.

There is no cure for high blood pressure. But the good news is the condition is both preventable and treatable. Adjustments to your lifestyle and, if necessary, medication can help you take control of your blood pressure and keep it at a safe level. Within these pages, you'll find practical advice you can put to use today to better manage your blood pressure. Much of the information is what Mayo Clinic doctors and other health care professionals use day in and day out in caring for their own patients.

About Mayo Clinic

Mayo Clinic pioneered the group practice of medicine. Today, with 2,000 physicians and scientists in virtually every medical specialty, Mayo Clinic is dedicated to providing comprehensive diagnosis, accurate answers and effective treatments for people with both common and uncommon medical conditions.

With this depth of medical knowledge, experience and expertise, Mayo Clinic occupies a unique position as a health information resource. Since 1983, Mayo Clinic has published reliable health information for millions of consumers through a variety of award-winning newsletters, books and online services. Look for information from Mayo Clinic to give you answers you can rely on for a healthier life. Revenue from our publishing activities supports Mayo Clinic programs, including medical education and medical research.

Editorial Staff

Editor-in-Chief
Sheldon G. Sheps, M.D.

Senior Editor
N. Nicole Spelhaug

Managing Editor
Karen R. Wallevand

Editorial Researcher
Brian M. Laing

Contributing Writers
Anne Christiansen
D. R. Martin
Stephen M. Miller
Susan Wichmann

Editorial Production
LeAnn M. Stee

Creative Director
Daniel W. Brevick

Graphic Designer
Kathryn K. Shepel

Medical Illustrators
John V. Hagen
Michael A. King

Editorial Assistants
Roberta J. Schwartz
Reneé Van Vleet
Sharon L. Wadleigh

Secretarial Assistance
Kathleen K. Iverson

Indexer
Larry Harrison

Reviewers and Contributors

Tammy F. Adams, R.N.
Kay M. Eberman, L.P.
Sharonne N. Hayes, M.D.
Donald D. Hensrud, M.D.
John E. Hodgson, L.P.
Ingeborg A. Hunder, R.N.
Richard D. Hurt, M.D.
Todd M. Johnson, R.Ph.
Thomas M. Kastner, M.D.

Ann Koranda, R.N.
Teresa K. Kubas, R.D.
Bruce Z. Morgenstern, M.D.
Carla Morrey, R.N.
Michael A. Morrey, Ph.D.
Jennifer K. Nelson, R.D.
John G. O'Meara, R.Ph.
Sandra J. Taler, M.D.

Preface

We believe that the more you know about high blood pressure, the more willing you'll be to take the necessary steps to lower your blood pressure and keep it under control. That's why we wrote this book.

The past 25 years have brought major advances in identifying and treating high blood pressure. Greater attention to this common illness is a major reason deaths from stroke have decreased approximately 60 percent and deaths from heart disease are down more than 50 percent.

Still, high blood pressure remains a serious problem. Of the 50 million Americans with the condition, only half are receiving treatment and only about a fourth have their blood pressure under control. This is disturbing considering that high blood pressure can almost always be successfully managed. And for people at risk, it often can be prevented.

In the pages that follow, you'll learn how high blood pressure develops and why it's so harmful if it's not controlled. We discuss the steps involved in diagnosing the disease and the factors taken into consideration in deciding how best to treat it. Most importantly, we give you practical tips and suggestions that you can use each day to help you manage your blood pressure. These include information on how to control your weight, improve your diet, increase your activity level, reduce your stress level and limit your use of tobacco, alcohol and caffeine. You'll also read about proper use of medications, monitoring your blood pressure at home and regular follow-up care. Plus, we address issues of concern to women and special at-risk populations.

Mayo Clinic physicians, nurses, registered dietitians, pharmacists and health educators reviewed the chapters to ensure you receive the latest and most accurate information.

This book, along with the advice of your personal physician, can help you live a longer, healthier life.

Sheldon G. Sheps, M.D.
Editor-in-Chief

Contents

Chapter 1	**Understanding High Blood Pressure**	11
	The basics of blood pressure	12
	What the numbers mean	15
	What's high blood pressure?	17
	Symptoms	18
	Complications	20
	Wrap-up	26
Chapter 2	**Are You at Risk?**	27
	Essential high blood pressure	27
	Risk factors	28
	Secondary high blood pressure	33
	Prevention	35
	Wrap-up	36
Chapter 3	**Diagnosis and Treatment**	37
	Measuring your blood pressure	38
	Receiving a diagnosis	39
	Getting an evaluation	40
	Deciding on treatment	45
	Becoming an active partner	48
	Wrap-up	50
Chapter 4	**Controlling Your Weight**	51
	Weight and blood pressure	51
	Overweight vs. obesity	52
	Finding your healthy weight	55
	Steps to successful weight loss	58
	Wrap-up	62
Chapter 5	**Getting More Active**	63
	Physical activity and blood pressure	63
	Activity vs. intensity	64
	What kind of activity?	65
	How much activity?	67
	A 6-step fitness plan	69

	Avoiding injury	75
	Wrap-up	76
Chapter 6	**Eating Well**	77
	The DASH study	77
	Basic principles of DASH	78
	How to eat with DASH	79
	A closer look at three important minerals	82
	A fresh approach to shopping	85
	Healthful cooking techniques	88
	Eating well when eating out	89
	Putting it all in perspective	91
	Wrap-up	92
Chapter 7	**The Shakedown on Salt**	93
	Sodium's role	93
	Sodium sensitivity	94
	Current recommendation	96
	The controversy	97
	What you should do	98
	Your sodium guide	101
	Wrap-up	106
Chapter 8	**Tobacco, Alcohol and Caffeine**	107
	Tobacco and high blood pressure	107
	Alcohol and high blood pressure	112
	Caffeine and high blood pressure	114
	Wrap-up	116
Chapter 9	**Managing Stress**	117
	What is stress?	118
	The stress response	118
	Stress and blood pressure	119
	Strategies for relieving stress	119
	Wrap-up	124
Chapter 10	**Medications and How They Work**	125
	The different types	126
	Diuretics	126
	Beta blockers	128

	ACE inhibitors	129
	Angiotensin II receptor blockers	130
	Calcium antagonists	131
	Alpha blockers	132
	Central-acting agents	133
	Direct vasodilators	134
	Emergency medications	134
	Combination drug therapy	135
	Finding the right medication	135
	A look ahead	137
	Wrap-up	138
Chapter 11	**Special Concerns**	139
	Issues for women	139
	High blood pressure in children	144
	High blood pressure in older adults	145
	High blood pressure and ethnic groups	145
	High blood pressure and other illnesses	146
	Difficult-to-control high blood pressure	149
	High blood pressure emergencies	150
	Wrap-up	152
Chapter 12	**Staying in Control**	153
	Home monitoring	153
	Using your medications wisely	158
	Getting regular follow-up care	164
	Reaching your goal	165
	Your family and friends	165
	A lifelong endeavor	166
	Wrap-up	166

Menus With DASH   *167*
High Blood Pressure Medications Guide   *182*
Index   *185*

Chapter 1

Understanding High Blood Pressure

Like many Americans, your blood pressure may be too high. That worries you, and that's why you're reading this book. Unfortunately, many people think that having high blood pressure isn't that big of a deal. It is.

High blood pressure is one of the leading causes of disability or death due to stroke, heart attack, heart failure and kidney failure. It's also the most common chronic illness Americans face. An estimated 50 million American adults have high blood pressure. That's about one out of every four people in this country. Each year, 2 million new cases of the disease are diagnosed.

However, high blood pressure often isn't given the serious attention it deserves. Nearly a third of the people affected by high blood pressure don't even know they have it. A major reason is that the disease generally doesn't produce any symptoms until it has progressed to an advanced stage.

Among people who are aware of their condition, only about half are getting treatment. And even fewer—only about a quarter of people with high blood pressure—have their blood pressure under control.

But there is good news. High blood pressure doesn't have to be deadly or disabling. The condition is easy to detect, and once you know you have it you can take steps to lower your blood pressure to a safe level. The two main methods for treating high blood pressure are changes in your lifestyle and medication.

You can live long and live well with high blood pressure. But you have to be willing to do your part and keep your blood pressure under control. Whether your high blood pressure was recently diagnosed, you've had it for many years or you simply want to prevent high blood pressure, this book can help you learn more about the disease. You'll also find out how your daily life affects your blood pressure and ways you can change bad habits into more healthful ones.

The basics of blood pressure

To better control your blood pressure, you need to know a few basics about the role of blood pressure and the organs and systems that help to regulate it. This information will make it easier to understand how high blood pressure develops and why it can be so harmful.

Your cardiovascular system

The explanation of blood pressure begins with your cardiovascular system, the system responsible for circulating blood through your heart and blood vessels (see illustration on opposite page).

With each beat of your heart, a surge of blood is released from your heart's main pumping chamber (left ventricle) into an intricate web of blood vessels that spread throughout your body.

Your arteries are the blood vessels that carry nutrients and oxygen-rich blood from your heart to your body's tissues and organs. The largest artery, called the aorta, is connected to the left ventricle and serves as the main channel for blood leaving your heart. The aorta branches off into smaller arteries, which turn into even smaller arteries, called arterioles.

Within your body's tissues and organs are microscopic blood vessels called capillaries. The capillaries exchange nutrients and fresh oxygen from the arterioles for carbon dioxide and other waste products produced by your cells. This spent, or "used," blood is sent back to your heart through a system of blood vessels called veins.

When it reaches your heart, blood from your veins is routed to your lungs, where it releases carbon dioxide and picks up a new supply of oxygen. This freshly oxygenated blood is sent back to your heart, ready to begin another journey. Other waste products are removed as your blood passes through your kidneys.

To keep this system working and all of the 11 pints of blood in your body moving, a certain amount of pressure is required. Your blood pressure is the force that's exerted on your artery walls as blood passes through. This force helps to keep blood in your arteries flowing smoothly.

Blood pressure is often compared to the pressure inside a garden hose. Without some type of force to push the water, it couldn't get from one end of the hose to the other.

Regulators of blood pressure

Several factors help control your blood pressure and keep it from increasing too high or decreasing too low. They include three major organs: your heart, your arteries and your kidneys.

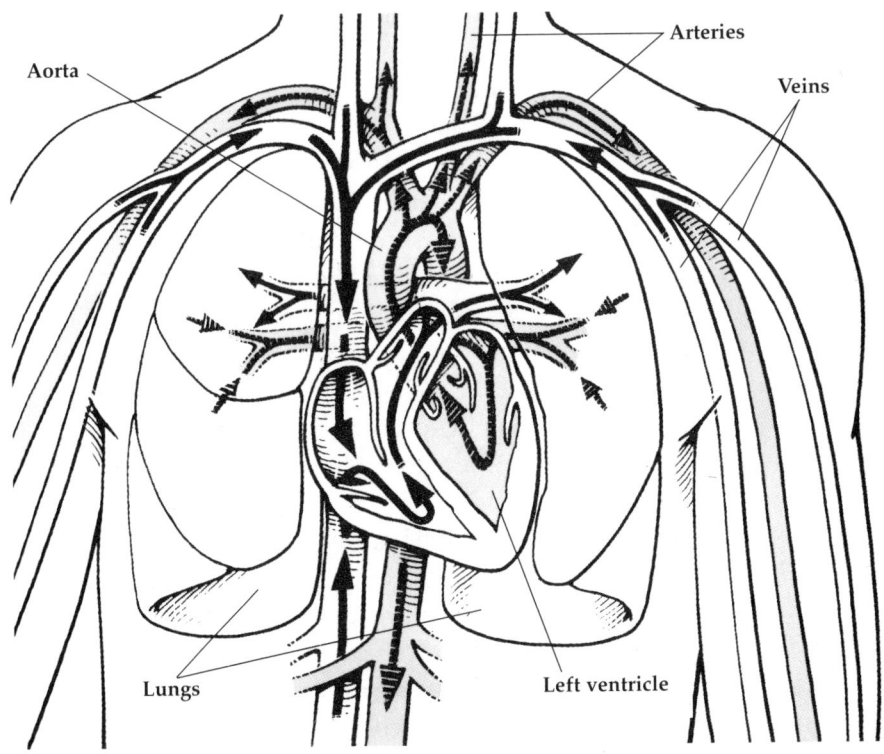

Each time your heart beats, blood is released from the left side of your heart (left ventricle) into the large blood vessel (aorta) that transports blood to your arteries. Blood returns to your heart through your veins. Before being circulated again, blood from your veins is sent to your lungs to load up on fresh oxygen.

Your heart. When your heart releases blood into your main artery (aorta), a certain amount of force is created by the pumping action of your heart muscle. The harder your heart muscle has to work to release the blood, the greater the force exerted on your arteries.

Your arteries. To accommodate the surge of blood coming from your heart, your arteries are lined with smooth muscles that allow them to expand and contract as blood courses through. The more "elastic" your arteries are, the less resistant they are to the flow of blood and the less force that's exerted on their walls. When arteries lose their elasticity or they become narrowed, resistance to blood flow increases and additional force is needed to push blood through the vessels.

Your kidneys. Your kidneys regulate the amount of sodium your body contains and the volume of water circulating in your body. Sodium retains water. Therefore, the more sodium that's in your body, the more water that's contained in your blood. This extra fluid can increase blood pressure. In addition, too much sodium can cause your blood vessels to narrow.

Other factors. Your central nervous system and many hormones and enzymes also influence your blood pressure. Within the walls of your heart and several blood vessels are tiny nodelike structures called baroreceptors. These structures work similar to the thermostat in your house. Baroreceptors continually monitor the pressure of blood through your arteries and veins. If they sense a change in pressure, they send signals to your brain to slow down or speed up your heart rate or to widen or narrow your arteries to keep your blood pressure within a normal range.

Your brain acts on messages from the baroreceptors by signaling the release of hormones and enzymes that affect the functioning of your heart, blood vessels and kidneys. One of the most significant hormones to affect blood pressure is the hormone epinephrine (EP-i-NEF-rin), also known as adrenaline. Epinephrine is released into your body during periods of high stress or tension, such as when you're frightened or while you're hurrying to complete a task on time.

Epinephrine causes your arteries to narrow and your heart contractions to become stronger and more rapid, increasing pressure in your arteries. People often refer to the release of epinephrine as being "pumped up" or on an "adrenaline high."

What the numbers mean

Your blood pressure is determined by measuring the pressure within your arteries. This is done with an instrument called a sphygmomanometer (SFIG-mo-mah-NOM-uh-tur). It includes an inflatable cuff that's wrapped around your upper arm, an air pump and column of mercury or a standardized pressure gauge. Blood pressure is expressed in terms of millimeters of mercury (mm Hg). The measurement refers to how high the pressure in your arteries can raise a column of mercury.

Two measurements

Two numbers are involved in a blood pressure reading. Both are important. The first of the two is your systolic pressure. This is the amount of pressure in your arteries when your heart contracts and releases blood into the aorta. The second number is your diastolic pressure. It tells how much pressure remains in your arteries between beats when your heart is relaxing and filling with blood. Your heart muscle must relax fully before it can contract again. During this time, your blood pressure decreases.

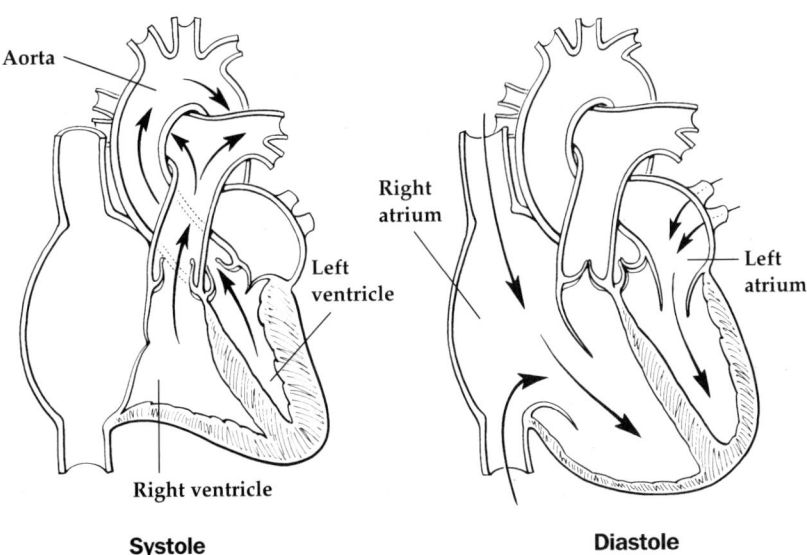

During systole (left), your heart muscle squeezes blood out of your heart's pumping chambers (ventricles). Blood on the right side of your heart goes to your lungs and that on the left side is pumped into the large blood vessel (aorta) that feeds your arteries. During diastole (right), your heart muscle relaxes and expands to allow blood to flow into the pumping chambers from your heart's holding chambers (atria).

The two numbers are usually written like a fraction: Systolic pressure is above or to the left and the diastolic pressure is below or to the right. When stated verbally, the word "over" is generally used to separate the two numbers.

At birth, your blood pressure is close to 90/60 mm Hg, or 90 "over" 60. During childhood, it slowly increases. Once you become an adult, the normal range of blood pressure extends from 120/80 mm Hg up to 139/89 mm Hg. However, systolic blood pressures between 130 and 139 mm Hg and diastolic pressures between 85 and 89 mm Hg are at the high end of what's considered a safe level. Readings within these ranges are often referred to as borderline or high-normal (see chart on opposite page).

An ideal or optimal blood pressure is 120/80 mm Hg or less. This is what you should aim for, if possible. If you're taking medication for high blood pressure, getting your blood pressure that low may not be reasonable or tolerable.

Daily ups and downs

A blood pressure reading reflects only what your blood pressure is at the moment it's measured. Throughout the day, your blood pressure naturally fluctuates. It increases during periods of activity when your heart has to work harder, such as when you exercise. And it decreases with rest when there's less demand on your heart, such as when you sleep. Your blood pressure also changes with changes in your body position, such as when you move from a lying or sitting to a standing position. Food, alcohol, pain, stress and strong emotions also increase your blood pressure. These daily ups and downs are perfectly normal.

Your blood pressure even changes with the time of day. Pressure in your arteries follows a natural fluctuation during a 24-hour period. It's usually the highest in the morning hours after you awaken and become active. It generally stays at about the same rate throughout the day and then late in the evening it begins to decrease. It reaches its lowest level in the early morning hours while you're sleeping. This 24-hour pattern is known as a circadian (SUR-kuh-DEE-un) rhythm. Your body has more than 100 circadian rhythms, each influencing a different body function.

If you're an evening or overnight shift worker, the circadian rhythm of your blood pressure is different and more closely aligned to your schedule of work and rest. That's because many circadian rhythms change with altered patterns of activity.

Getting an accurate reading

To get a good indication of what your average blood pressure is, the best time to measure it is during the day after you've been active for a few hours. If you exercise in the morning, it's better to measure your blood pressure beforehand or several hours afterward. After physical activity, your blood pressure stays at a temporary low level for 1 to 2 hours. Readings taken during this time may not reflect your average pressure.

You also shouldn't smoke or drink caffeine or alcohol 30 minutes before measuring your blood pressure. Tobacco and caffeine can temporarily increase your pressure. Alcohol may temporarily decrease your blood pressure. In some people, though, alcohol has the opposite effect. It increases blood pressure. In addition, you should wait 5 minutes after you sit down before taking a reading so your blood pressure has time to adjust to your change in position and activity.

Classification of high blood pressure

	Systolic (mm Hg)		Diastolic (mm Hg)
Optimal*	120 or less	and	80 or less
Normal	129 or less	and	84 or less
High-normal	130-139	or	85-89
Hypertension			
Stage 1†	140-159	or	90-99
Stage 2†	160-179	or	100-109
Stage 3†	180 or higher	or	110 or higher

*Optimal pressure with respect to cardiovascular risk.
†Based on the average of two or more readings taken at each of two or more visits after an initial screening.
From National Institutes of Health. The Sixth Report of the Joint National Committee on Prevention, Detection, Evaluation, and Treatment of High Blood Pressure, 1997.

What's high blood pressure?

When the complex system that regulates your blood pressure doesn't work as it's supposed to, too much pressure can develop within your arteries. Increased pressure in your arteries that continues on a persistent basis is called high blood pressure.

The medical term for the condition is hypertension, meaning high tension in your arteries. Hypertension doesn't mean nervous tension, as many people often believe. You can be a calm, relaxed person and still have high blood pressure.

Your blood pressure is considered high if your systolic pressure is consistently 140 mm Hg or higher, your diastolic pressure is consistently 90 mm Hg or higher, or both.

There are three separate stages of high blood pressure, based on increasing severity. They're referred to simply as stages 1, 2 and 3. The terms "mild" and "moderate" are no longer used to define levels of high blood pressure to avoid the possibility that people will mistakenly believe mild or moderate high blood pressure isn't serious.

High blood pressure generally develops slowly. In most instances, people start out with normal blood pressure that progresses to borderline (high-normal) blood pressure and, eventually, to stage 1 high blood pressure. Among people whose blood pressure is uncontrolled, most—almost 75 percent—have stage 1 high blood pressure. About 20 percent of people have stage 2 disease, and about 5 percent have stage 3 high blood pressure.

Left untreated, the excessive force of your blood can damage many of your body's organs and tissues. The higher your blood pressure stage, the greater the risk that injury will occur. However, even stage 1 high blood pressure can be harmful if it continues over a period of several months to years.

When coupled with other factors known to be detrimental to your health, such as obesity or tobacco use, your risk for injury from high blood pressure is even greater.

Symptoms

High blood pressure is often called the "silent killer" because it doesn't produce any signs or symptoms to warn you that you have a problem.

People often think that headaches, dizziness or nosebleeds are common warning signs of high blood pressure. It's true that a few people with early-stage high blood pressure have a dull ache in the back of their head when they wake in the morning. Or, perhaps they have a few more nosebleeds than normal. But generally, most people don't experience any signs or symptoms.

When your blood pressure drops too low

Generally, the lower your blood pressure reading, the better. But in some cases, your blood pressure can drop too low, just as it can rise too high. Low blood pressure, called hypotension, can be life-threatening if it falls to dangerously low levels. However, this is rare.

Chronic low blood pressure—blood pressure that's below normal but not hazardously so—is fairly common. It can result from various factors, including medications to treat high blood pressure and complications of diabetes. The middle stage (second trimester) of pregnancy also can cause below-normal blood pressure.

A potentially dangerous side effect of chronic low blood pressure is postural hypotension. It's a condition in which you feel dizzy or faint when you stand too quickly.

When you stand, the force of gravity causes blood to pool in your legs, which produces a sudden drop in blood pressure. Normally, the system that regulates your blood pressure counteracts the decrease almost simultaneously by narrowing your blood vessels and increasing the volume of blood flow from your heart. As a result, when you change positions, you don't experience any symptoms.

But if your blood pressure is chronically low, it takes longer for your body to respond to the change in pressure when you stand. Postural hypotension also tends to become more common with advanced age as nerve signals and regulatory system responses become slowed. The danger is, if you become too dizzy or lose consciousness, you can fall and injure yourself.

You can generally avoid this problem by standing more slowly and holding on to something while you stand. Also, wait a few seconds after standing and before walking so your body has time to adjust to the pressure change. Crossing your legs and squeezing your thighs together (like a scissors) after standing also may help by reducing blood flow to your legs.

However, see your doctor if you experience persistent dizziness or fainting. You may have another health condition that's causing these symptoms or that's making your symptoms worse than usual.

You can have high blood pressure for years without ever knowing it. In fact, about 15 million Americans right now have no idea that their blood pressure is too high. The condition is most often discovered during a routine physical examination when a doctor or nurse measures your blood pressure.

Signs and symptoms such as headaches, dizziness or nosebleeds typically don't occur until high blood pressure has advanced to a higher, and possibly life-threatening, stage. However, even some people with stage 3 high blood pressure don't experience any signs or symptoms.

Other symptoms sometimes associated with high blood pressure, such as excessive perspiration, muscle cramps, weakness, frequent urination or rapid or irregular heartbeats (palpitations), generally are caused by other conditions that can lead to uncontrolled high blood pressure.

Complications

High blood pressure needs to be controlled because, over time, the excessive force on your artery walls can seriously damage many of your body's vital organs. Generally, the higher your high blood pressure or the longer it goes uncontrolled, the greater the damage. And again, by the time symptoms appear, injury may have already occurred.

Many studies have demonstrated a direct relationship between uncontrolled high blood pressure and increased risk for stroke, heart attack and heart and kidney failure. Sites in your body typically most affected by high blood pressure include your arteries, heart, brain, kidneys and eyes.

Your arteries

Damage to your arteries from high blood pressure can result in arteriosclerosis, atherosclerosis and aneurysm.

Arteriosclerosis. Healthy arteries are like healthy muscles. They're flexible, strong and elastic. Their inside lining is smooth so that blood can flow through them unrestricted. But over a period of years, too much pressure in your arteries can make the walls thick and stiff.

The term arteriosclerosis (ahr-TEER-ee-o-skluh-RO-sis) means hardening of your arteries. It comes from the Greek word "sklerosis," for hardening. Sometimes, stiffened arteries in your forearms can actually be felt, and they may resemble small, hard pipes.

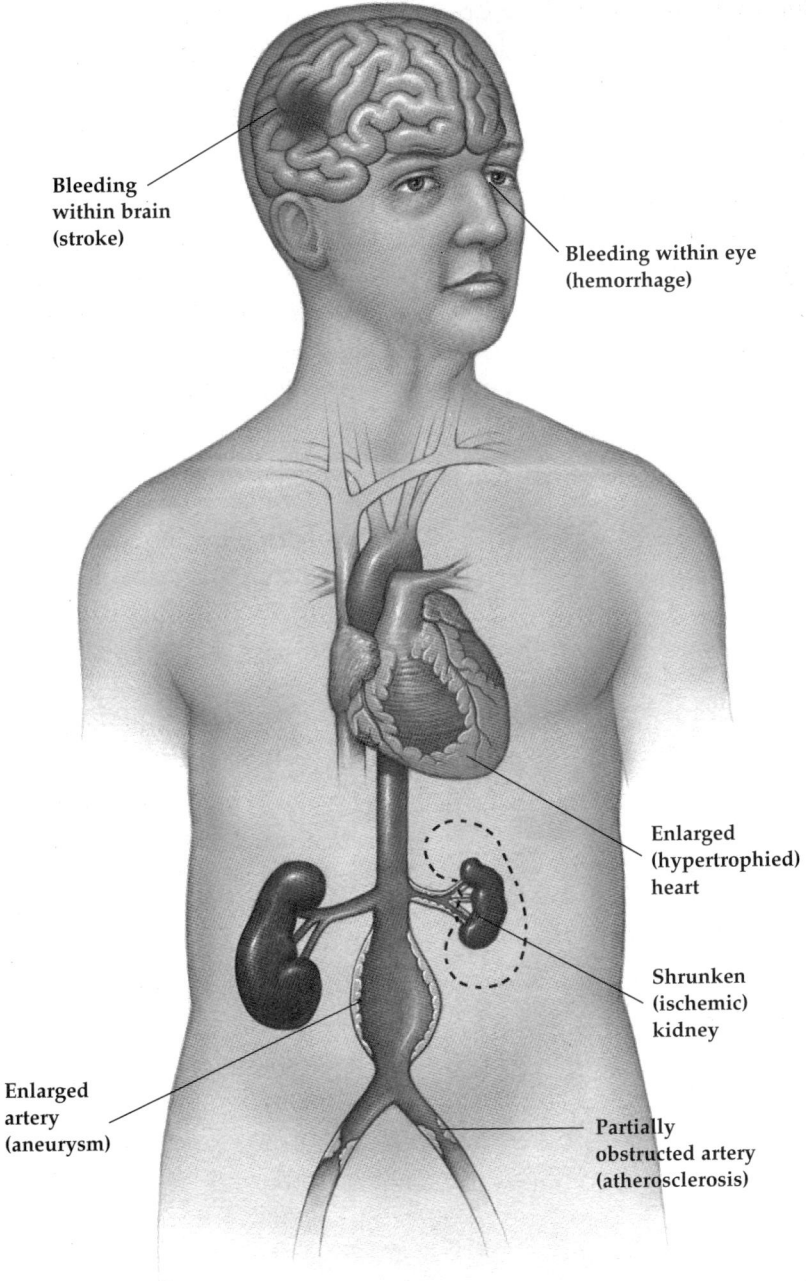

Left untreated, high blood pressure can damage tissues and organs throughout your body. Sites in your body most affected by high blood pressure include your arteries, heart, brain, kidneys and eyes.

Atherosclerosis. High blood pressure can accelerate the accumulation of fatty deposits in and under the lining of artery walls. The name atherosclerosis (ATH-ur-o-skluh-RO-sis) comes from the Greek word "ather," meaning porridge, because the fatty deposits are soft and resemble porridge.

When the inner wall of an artery is damaged, blood cells called platelets often clump at the injury site. In addition, fat deposits also gather at the site. Initially, the deposits are only streaks of fat-containing cells. But, as the deposits accumulate they invade some of the deeper layers of your artery walls, causing the walls to become scarred. Large accumulations of fatty deposits are called plaque. Over time, plaque can harden.

The greatest danger from formation of plaque is the narrowing of the channel through which your blood flows. When this happens, organs and tissues that an artery supplies blood to don't receive their full quota. Your body responds to the shortage of blood by increasing blood pressure to maintain adequate blood flow. The increase in blood pressure leads to further blood vessel damage, and thus a vicious cycle is set in motion. In addition, a plaque may break apart and block the artery, causing a blood clot, or travel with your blood until it lodges in a smaller artery.

Arteriosclerosis and atherosclerosis can occur in arteries anywhere within your body, but the diseases most often affect arteries in your heart, brain and kidneys.

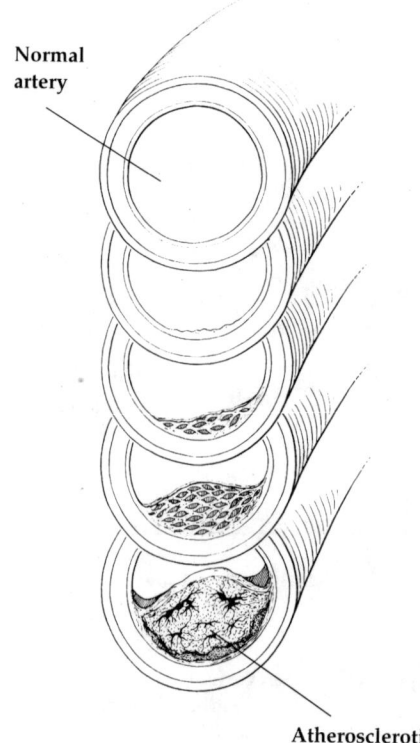

Normal artery

Atherosclerotic plaque

In atherosclerosis, plaque deposits gradually accumulate in the lining of your arteries. As the deposits enlarge, blood circulation decreases and blood pressure increases. This increases your risk for heart attack, stroke and other vascular problems.

Aneurysm. When a blood vessel loses elasticity and weakens, a spot in its wall may bulge or balloon. Aneurysms most commonly occur in a brain artery or in the lower portion of your aorta that passes through your abdomen. The danger with any aneurysm is that it may leak or burst, causing life-threatening bleeding.

In their early stages, aneurysms generally don't produce any symptoms. In more advanced stages, an aneurysm in a brain artery can lead to a severe headache that doesn't go away. An advanced abdominal aneurysm may cause constant pain in your abdomen or lower back. Occasionally, during a physical examination, a doctor can detect an abdominal aneurysm by feeling the pulsating vessel while pressing lightly on your abdomen.

The sooner high blood pressure is controlled, the less chance that these blood vessel diseases will occur or become severe.

Your heart

High blood pressure can damage your heart in three significant ways.

Coronary artery disease. The major cause of death in people with uncontrolled high blood pressure is one or more complications of coronary artery disease. Coronary artery disease refers to damage to the major arteries (coronary) feeding your heart muscle. Accumulation of plaque in these arteries is common among people with high blood pressure. The plaque reduces the flow of blood to your heart muscle, which can lead to a heart attack if your heart muscle is deprived of too much blood.

Left ventricular hypertrophy. Blood pressure is like a weight or load that your heart muscle must lift. When your heart pumps blood into your aorta, it has to push the blood out against the pressure inside your arteries. The higher the pressure, the harder the muscle has to work. And like any muscle, the harder your heart muscle works, the larger it gets.

Eventually, your heart can't keep up with the excessive workload, and the muscular wall of its main pumping chamber (left ventricle) starts to thicken (hypertrophy). As the ventricle enlarges, it requires an increased supply of blood. But because high blood pressure also causes blood vessels feeding your heart to narrow, the vessels often can't supply enough blood to meet your heart's needs. Left ventricular hypertrophy is associated with a higher risk of sudden death and heart attack.

Heart failure. When your heart muscle enlarges, it can weaken and become less efficient. Basically, it requires more strength to pump less blood. This can lead to heart failure. In this condition, your heart isn't able to pump the blood returning to it fast enough. As a result, fluid can back up and start to accumulate in your lungs, legs and other tissues.

Accumulation of fluid is called edema (uh-DEE-muh). When fluid collects in your lungs, it leads to shortness of breath. Buildup of fluid in your legs causes your feet and ankles to swell.

Controlling high blood pressure for a period of 5 or more years greatly reduces your risk for these cardiovascular diseases. Your risk for a heart attack decreases by about 20 percent, and your risk for heart failure declines by more than 50 percent.

Your brain

High blood pressure significantly increases your odds for having a stroke. In fact, high blood pressure is the most important risk factor for stroke. It's estimated that 70 percent of all strokes occur in people with high blood pressure.

A stroke, also called a brain attack, is a type of brain injury caused by a blocked or ruptured blood vessel in your brain that disturbs your brain's blood supply. There are two main types of stroke: ischemic (is-KEEM-ik) and hemorrhagic (HEM-uh-RAJ-ik).

Ischemic strokes. These strokes are the most common, accounting for about 80 percent of all strokes. They result from a blood clot due to accumulation of plaque in an artery. The plaque roughens the inside of the blood vessel surface, forcing blood to flow around the plaque, which can trigger development of a blood clot. More than half of ischemic strokes are caused by stationary (thrombotic) blood clots that develop in the arteries leading from your heart to your brain. The arteries in your neck (carotid) are the most common locations for development of a clot.

A less frequent form of ischemic stroke occurs when a tiny piece of clotted blood breaks loose from an artery wall and is swept through larger arteries into smaller vessels in your brain. A clot that may have developed in a chamber in your heart can also break loose. If the moving (embolic) clot lodges in a small artery and blocks blood flow to a portion of your brain, a stroke occurs.

Ischemic strokes usually affect the portion of your brain that controls your movement, language and senses, called the cerebrum.

Hemorrhagic strokes. This type of stroke occurs when a blood vessel in your brain leaks or ruptures. Blood from the hemorrhage spills into surrounding brain tissue, damaging the tissue. Brain cells beyond the leak or rupture are also damaged because they're deprived of blood.

One cause of a hemorrhagic stroke is an aneurysm. A small tear in a brain artery also can cause blood to leak. Hemorrhagic strokes are less common, but they're more deadly.

The good news is that improved detection and treatment of high blood pressure during the past 25 years have contributed to a dramatic reduction in the number of strokes. When your blood pressure is lowered through appropriate treatment, your risk for stroke decreases remarkably—about 40 percent over a period of 2 to 5 years.

In addition, clot-busting medications given within the first few hours after symptoms of an ischemic stroke begin can greatly reduce disability from a stroke.

Your kidneys

About one-fifth of the blood pumped by your heart goes to your kidneys. Tiny filtering structures in your kidneys called nephrons filter out waste products in your blood, which are later excreted in your urine. Your kidneys also control the balance of minerals, acids and water in your blood. High blood pressure can interfere with this intricate process, eventually causing your kidneys to fail.

When blood vessels in your kidneys become weakened or narrowed due to high blood pressure, blood flow to the nephrons is reduced and your kidneys can't eliminate all of the waste products in your blood. Over time, waste can build up in your blood and your kidneys can shrink and quit functioning. High blood pressure and diabetes are the most common causes of kidney failure.

When your kidneys stop functioning, you need to undergo kidney dialysis, and you may need a kidney transplant. Kidney dialysis is a process by which waste products in your blood are filtered out by a machine. A surgeon creates an access point for blood to leave and reenter your body during dialysis. Usually, the access is in the forearm.

Because part of the role of your kidneys is to help control blood pressure by regulating the amount of sodium and water in your blood, damage to your kidneys can worsen your high blood pressure. This can produce a destructive cycle that, ultimately, results in increasing blood pressure and a gradual failure of your kidneys to remove impurities from your blood.

Control of high blood pressure can reduce progression from kidney damage to kidney failure.

Your eyes
High blood pressure speeds the normal aging of tiny blood vessels in your eyes. In severe cases, it may even lead to vision loss.

Occasionally, a simple eye examination will trigger the discovery of high blood pressure. Shining a light into your eye makes tiny blood vessels in the back of your eye (retina) visible. In the early stages of high blood pressure, these blood vessels can thicken and narrow. Eventually, the vessels can develop blockages and they can compress nearby veins, interfering with blood flow in the veins.

High blood pressure also can cause tiny blood vessels in your retina to tear and leak blood and fluid into surrounding tissue. In severe cases, the nerve that carries visual signals from your retina to your brain (optic nerve) may start to swell. This can result in a loss of vision.

Injury to arteries in your retina is a good indication that blood vessels elsewhere in your body also have been damaged.

Early treatment can generally prevent eye complications.

Wrap-up

Key points to remember from this chapter:
- Blood pressure is necessary for smooth flow of blood through your heart and blood vessels.
- Both numbers in a blood pressure reading are equally important.
- High blood pressure refers to systolic blood pressure that's consistently 140 mm Hg or higher, diastolic pressure that's consistently 90 mm Hg or higher, or both.
- An estimated 50 million Americans have high blood pressure, but only about a quarter have their disease under control.
- High blood pressure is often called the silent killer because it typically doesn't produce any symptoms.
- Left untreated, high blood pressure can lead to stroke, heart attack, heart failure and kidney failure.
- By controlling high blood pressure, you significantly reduce your risk for disability or death related to the disease.

Chapter 2

Are You at Risk?

With any disease, you naturally want to know what causes it. What makes it occur in some people but not in others? Unfortunately, with high blood pressure, the reason the condition develops is unknown in most people.

However, it's clear that certain factors can put you at greater risk for high blood pressure. By knowing what these factors are, you can take steps to minimize your risk and possibly prevent the disease from occurring.

Essential high blood pressure

There are two forms of high blood pressure: essential and secondary. Essential is the most common. Approximately 95 percent of people with high blood pressure have essential disease, also known as primary high blood pressure.

Essential high blood pressure differs from secondary high blood pressure in that it has no obvious cause. Among the large majority of people who have high blood pressure, it's difficult to pinpoint exactly what's triggering the increase in their blood pressure.

Researchers are studying the possibility that your genes are responsible for the development of high blood pressure. But it's doubtful they'll be able to link a specific genetic defect to all essential

disease. More likely, essential high blood pressure results from a combination of factors related to:
- Motion (widening and narrowing) of your blood vessels
- Increased fluid in your blood
- Functioning of your blood flow sensors (baroreceptors)
- Production of chemicals that influence how your blood vessels function
- Secretion of hormones
- Volume of blood pumped by your heart
- Nerve control of your cardiovascular system

Risk factors

Certain genetic traits or lifestyle habits play an important role in the development of essential high blood pressure. Generally, the more of these risk factors you have, the greater the odds that you'll have high blood pressure during your lifetime. Most risk factors you can control, others you can't.

Unmodifiable risk factors

There are four major risk factors for high blood pressure that you can't control.

Race. High blood pressure occurs almost two times more frequently in blacks of African-American descent than in whites. The highest rates of high blood pressure in the United States are among blacks living in the southeastern states.

High blood pressure generally develops at an earlier age in blacks. Plus, it's usually more severe and tends to progress more rapidly. These are major reasons blacks have the highest death rate from complications related to the disease.

Among some populations of American Indians, the prevalence of high blood pressure is also higher than in whites. Among Hispanics, high blood pressure is slightly less common than in whites.

Age. Your risk for high blood pressure increases with your age. Although high blood pressure can occur at any age, it's most often detected in people age 35 or older. Among Americans age 65 or older, more than half have high blood pressure.

It's fairly common for your blood pressure to increase slightly with age. This is often due to natural changes in your body affecting your heart, blood vessels and hormones. However, when these changes are coupled with other risk factors, they can lead to the development of high blood pressure.

Family history. High blood pressure tends to run in families. If one of your parents has high blood pressure you have about a 25 percent chance of developing it during your lifetime. If both your mother and father have high blood pressure, you have about a 60 percent chance of acquiring the disease.

Studies of twins and of people within the same family who have high blood pressure show that an inherited (genetic) component may play a role in some cases of the disease. One theory being investigated has to do with the hormone angiotensin (AN-jee-oh-TEN-sin). When it reaches your bloodstream, the hormone is converted into a substance called angiotensin II, which constricts your blood vessels and causes your kidneys to retain water and sodium. Researchers believe that in some people with high blood pressure, the gene that determines your body's production and release of angiotensin may be flawed, causing your body to produce too much.

However, just because high blood pressure commonly exists in your family doesn't mean you're destined to get it. Even in families in which high blood pressure is prevalent, some blood relatives never develop the disease.

Sex. Among young and middle-aged adults, men are more likely to have high blood pressure than women. Later on, the reverse is true. After about age 50, when most women are beyond menopause, high blood pressure becomes more common in women than in men.

Modifiable risk factors
These are risk factors for high blood pressure that you can control.

Obesity. Being overweight increases your risk for development of high blood pressure for several reasons. The more body mass you have, the more blood you need to supply oxygen and nutrients to your tissues. That means the volume of blood being circulated through your blood vessels is increased, creating extra force on your artery walls.

Excess weight also can increase your heart rate and the level of insulin in your blood. Increased insulin causes your body to retain sodium and water.

In addition, some people who are overweight follow a diet that's too high in fat, especially saturated and trans fats. These fats promote the accumulation of fatty deposits (plaque) in your arteries, causing narrowing of your arteries. Your diet contains too much fat if more than 30 percent of your total daily calories come from fat.

Inactivity. Lack of physical activity increases your risk for high blood pressure by increasing your risk for becoming overweight. People who are inactive also tend to have higher heart rates and their heart muscle has to work harder with each contraction. The harder and more often your heart has to pump, the greater the force being exerted on your arteries.

The fattening of America

America's waistline is expanding. An estimated 97 million adults are either overweight or obese. That's more than half of the adult population. Excess weight is now the second leading cause of preventable death in the United States, led only by smoking.

Latest results from the Third National Health and Nutrition Examination Survey (NHANES III) show that between 1960 and 1994 adults in the United States who were overweight increased from 30.5 percent to 32 percent. During the same period, obese adults increased from 12.8 percent to 22.5 percent.

You're more likely to become overweight or obese as you get older. According to the latest figures, 73 percent of all men age 50 or older and 65 percent of all women age 50 or older are overweight or obese. Overweight is defined as a body mass index (BMI) of 25 to 29. Obesity is defined as a BMI of 30 or greater. Body mass index is discussed in Chapter 4 (page 52).

And it's not just adults who are gaining weight. According to the NHANES III figures, almost 14 percent of children and 11.5 percent of adolescents are overweight. Other studies suggest these figures may be even higher.

A combination of factors, including genes, an inactive lifestyle, consuming too many calories and easy access to food, may be responsible for this growing problem.

Tobacco use. The chemicals in tobacco can damage the lining of your artery walls, making them more prone to the accumulation of plaque.

Nicotine in tobacco also makes your heart work harder by temporarily constricting your blood vessels and increasing your heart rate and blood pressure. These effects occur because of increased hormone production during tobacco use, including increased levels of the hormone epinephrine (adrenaline).

In addition, carbon monoxide in cigarette smoke replaces oxygen in your blood. This can increase blood pressure by forcing your heart to work harder to supply adequate oxygen to your body's organs and tissues.

Sodium sensitivity. Your body needs a certain amount of the mineral sodium to maintain the chemistry that occurs within your cells. A common source of sodium is table salt (sodium chloride), which is composed of about 40 percent sodium and 60 percent chloride.

However, some people's bodies are more sensitive to the presence of sodium in their blood than others. People who are sodium-sensitive retain sodium more easily, leading to fluid retention and increased blood pressure. If you're among this group, excessive sodium in your diet can increase your chances for having high blood pressure.

More than a third of Americans with high blood pressure may be sodium-sensitive. Among blacks, the percentage is even higher. As you age, your sensitivity to sodium often becomes more pronounced.

Low potassium. Potassium is a mineral that helps balance the amount of sodium in cell fluids. It gets rid of excess sodium in your cells by way of your kidneys, which filter out the sodium to be excreted in your urine.

If your diet doesn't include enough potassium, or your body isn't able to retain a proper amount, too much sodium can accumulate, increasing your risk for development of high blood pressure.

Excessive alcohol. People who have three or more drinks a day have a greater incidence of high blood pressure than people who don't drink alcohol or who have less than three drinks daily. Excessive alcohol use contributes to about 8 percent of all cases of high blood pressure.

Exactly how or why alcohol increases blood pressure isn't fully understood. But it's known that, over time, heavy drinking can damage your heart muscle.

Stress. Stress doesn't cause persistent high blood pressure. But high levels of stress can lead to a temporary, but dramatic, increase in blood pressure. If these temporary episodes occur often enough, over time they can damage your blood vessels, heart and kidneys in the same manner as persistent high blood pressure.

Stress also can promote high blood pressure by causing you to develop unhealthful habits known to increase your risk for the disease. Some people bothered by stress turn to smoking, alcohol or food (usually fatty or salty foods) to relieve their stress.

Other illnesses
You also may be at increased risk for development of high blood pressure if you have a chronic illness. Illnesses that can contribute to increased blood pressure or make high blood pressure more difficult to control are described here.

High cholesterol. High levels of cholesterol, a fat-like substance in your blood, promote the development of plaque in your arteries, causing your arteries to narrow. Narrowed arteries (atherosclerosis) can increase your blood pressure.

Diabetes. Too much sugar in your blood can damage many of your organs and tissues, leading to atherosclerosis, kidney disease and coronary artery disease. These diseases all affect your blood pressure.

Sleep apnea. This severe form of snoring that interrupts your breathing while you sleep can stress your heart and increase your risk for development of high blood pressure.

Heart failure. If your heart muscle is damaged or weakened, possibly due to a heart attack, it has to work harder to pump blood. High blood pressure that's uncontrolled increases demand on your weakened heart and complicates the treatment of both conditions.

A multiplying effect
Risk factors usually don't function independently. They often interact with each other in important ways. For example, if you have two risk factors—you're overweight and you're inactive—your odds of having high blood pressure are much higher than if you had either one alone.

By the same token, working to reduce one risk factor may have benefits for others. Your total reduction in risk may be more than the sum of that one factor alone.

Remember: Risk refers to odds or chances, not to inevitability or guarantees. Clearly, risk factors affect your chances for having high blood pressure. But having one or more risk factors doesn't guarantee that you'll get high blood pressure, just as having no risk factors doesn't guarantee that you won't.

Secondary high blood pressure

Secondary high blood pressure refers to high blood pressure that has a known cause. Doctors are able to identify an underlying illness or condition that's triggering your blood pressure to increase. This form of high blood pressure occurs infrequently, affecting only about 5 percent of people with increased blood pressure.

As opposed to essential high blood pressure, which doctors can treat but not cure, secondary high blood pressure often can be cured. Once the underlying disease or condition is corrected, blood pressure typically decreases. In many people, their blood pressure returns to normal.

Causes

The following are illnesses and conditions that can lead to secondary high blood pressure. They differ from the illnesses listed on the previous page in that they can actually cause high blood pressure, not just increase your risk for it.

Kidney disease. Your kidneys are one of the main regulators of your blood pressure. If a condition or illness, such as an injury, inflammation or the development of fluid-filled sacs (cysts), causes your kidneys to quit functioning normally, your blood pressure can increase.

Adrenal disease. Your adrenal glands make hormones, including the hormones epinephrine (adrenaline), norepinephrine (noradrenaline), aldosterone and cortisol, that help regulate your blood pressure and heart rate. Overgrowth of your adrenal cells or development of a tumor that affects release of these hormones into your bloodstream can lead to high blood pressure.

Thyroid disease. Hormones made by your thyroid gland regulate all aspects of your metabolism, from the rate at which your heart beats to the speed at which you burn calories. When your thyroid gland releases excessive amounts of hormones (hyperthyroidism), your heart rate speeds up and demands on your cardiovascular system are increased. This extra strain can lead to the development of high blood pressure.

Interestingly, a decrease in thyroid hormones (hypothyroidism) can also cause high blood pressure. The condition is thought to increase blood pressure by increasing fluid retention.

Blood vessel abnormalities. In rare cases, secondary high blood pressure can result from a birth defect in which your aorta narrows after it branches off into the arteries that lead to your neck and arms. Blood pressures in the upper parts of your body are high, but those in your abdomen and legs are lower. This defect (coarctation) most often occurs in young people with high blood pressure.

Secondary high blood pressure also can result from narrowing of one or both of the arteries leading to your kidneys. The narrowing causes release of the hormone renin (REE-nin), which increases blood pressure. The condition may result from accumulation of plaque or an abnormality that causes the middle layer of an artery wall to become too thick. This form of artery wall thickening, called fibromuscular dysplasia, occurs more often in women than men.

Pregnancy. During the last 3 months (third trimester) of pregnancy, a small percentage of pregnant women develop a condition called preeclampsia. It's characterized by a significant increase in blood pressure, swelling and excess protein in your urine. After the baby is born, your blood pressure usually returns to normal.

Preeclampsia is discussed further in Chapter 11 (page 142).

Medications. Birth control pills may increase a woman's blood pressure very slightly. In a few cases, though, the increase may be more dramatic, triggering the development of high blood pressure.

Several other drugs can also increase blood pressure in some people. They include over-the-counter products such as cold remedies, nasal decongestants, appetite suppressants and nonsteroidal anti-inflammatory drugs (NSAIDs), as well as prescription medications, including steroids, tricyclic antidepressants, cyclosporine and erythropoietin.

Illicit drug use. Illegal drugs, such as cocaine and amphetamines, can lead to high blood pressure by damaging your heart muscle, narrowing the arteries that supply blood to your heart or increasing your heart rate.

Prevention

High blood pressure is often preventable. And greater efforts are now being made within the medical community to prevent the disease, as well as treat it. These efforts are aimed mainly at people with borderline (high-normal) blood pressure.

For years, as long as your blood pressure was below the cutoff for being high, it was considered OK. That's not true anymore. Doctors now know that high-normal blood pressure often leads to high blood pressure. And they've found that even high-normal blood pressure may increase your risk for cardiovascular disease.

High-normal blood pressure refers to persistent systolic readings between 130 and 139 mm Hg, diastolic readings between 85 and 89 mm Hg, or both. If your blood pressure is within these ranges, you should take steps to lower it until it reaches a normal or, ideally, optimal level (see page 17).

You can reduce your blood pressure by eliminating or changing those risk factors that you can control. That may include:
- Losing weight, if you're overweight
- Becoming more physically active
- Eating more healthfully
- Quitting smoking
- Limiting alcohol

Why act now?
You may wonder why it's so important to prevent high blood pressure. Why not simply wait for it to develop and then treat it?

It's true that most people at risk for high blood pressure don't make changes in their lifestyle until after their blood pressures have gotten too high. But there are many reasons why it's better to act early instead of later.

Better odds. Generally, the younger you are when you try to change your lifestyle, the better your chances of succeeding. The longer you're involved in an unhealthful habit, the more difficult it is for you to change that habit.

Reduced health risks. Even if you're able to control your high blood pressure after the disease develops, you still have a higher risk of a heart attack or stroke than people who don't have high blood pressure.

Control difficulties. Managing high blood pressure isn't always easy. Only about a quarter of Americans with high blood pressure have their condition under control.

Side effects. Medications to treat high blood pressure can sometimes cause side effects, such as fatigue, headaches, constipation, a nagging cough and loss of sex drive.

Cost. Treating high blood pressure typically includes more frequent trips to your doctor. Plus, you may need to take medication daily.

Wrap-up

Key points to remember from this chapter:
- There are two forms of high blood pressure: essential (primary) and secondary. The cause of essential high blood pressure, the most common type, isn't known. Secondary high blood pressure results from an underlying illness or condition. This form of high blood pressure is often curable.
- Certain genetic traits or lifestyle factors place you at increased risk for the development of high blood pressure. Generally, the more of them you have, the greater your risk.
- You may be able to prevent high blood pressure by eliminating or modifying risk factors that you can change.
- If you have borderline (high-normal) blood pressure, reducing it to a normal or optimal level can keep you from developing high blood pressure.

Chapter 3

Diagnosis and Treatment

Unlike many other health conditions, high blood pressure rarely produces any signs or symptoms to warn you that something's wrong. Most people who have uncontrolled high blood pressure feel and look just fine.

That's why it's important to have your blood pressure checked at least every 2 years. Otherwise, you could be living with increased blood pressure for years and never know it.

It's during a routine medical appointment that most people first learn their blood pressure is too high. Fortunately, diagnosing high blood pressure is a relatively simple and straightforward process. It involves having your blood pressure measured periodically over a period of a few weeks to months to see if it remains increased.

Your doctor will also ask you questions about your health and your family's health, do a physical examination and have you undergo some routine tests. These steps are done to make sure your organs haven't been damaged and to prevent additional health problems associated with high blood pressure. Results from the history, examination and tests are also important in deciding how best to treat your condition.

The two methods for reducing and controlling high blood pressure are lifestyle changes and medication. Whether you'll need medication depends on your blood pressure stage, your risk for other health problems and whether the disease has caused any organ damage.

Measuring your blood pressure

Determining your blood pressure levels is a fairly easy procedure. Here's how a measurement is taken.

A sphygmomanometer is the device that measures blood pressure. It includes an inflatable arm cuff with an attached air pump and a column of mercury or a standardized pressure gauge.

During a blood pressure measurement, the cuff is wrapped around your upper arm. Air is then pumped into the cuff by squeezing the bulb on the air pump. The cuff is inflated until the pressure inside it reaches a level well above your systolic pressure (upper number). This causes the main artery in your arm (brachial artery) to collapse, cutting off blood flow to the rest of your arm. When the artery collapses, no sounds are heard through a stethoscope that's placed over the artery, just below the cuff.

Air is then slowly released from the cuff, gradually reducing pressure on the artery. As soon as pressure in the cuff equals your systolic pressure, blood begins to spurt through your artery again. This causes a thumping sound to be heard through the stethoscope. The number on the mercury column or air pressure gauge that coincides with the moment you first hear the return of blood flow is your systolic pressure.

As air continues to be released from the cuff, pressure on the brachial artery drops further. When the artery is fully open again, the thumping sounds become inaudible. The reading on the mercury column or pressure gauge at the moment the sounds disappear is equivalent to your diastolic pressure (lower number).

Newer, electronic sphygmomanometers work in a similar fashion, but they include a monitor that's fully automatic. It inflates and deflates the cuff, detects your systolic and diastolic pressures and then displays your measurements on a digital screen. These devices are discussed in more detail in Chapter 12 (page 154).

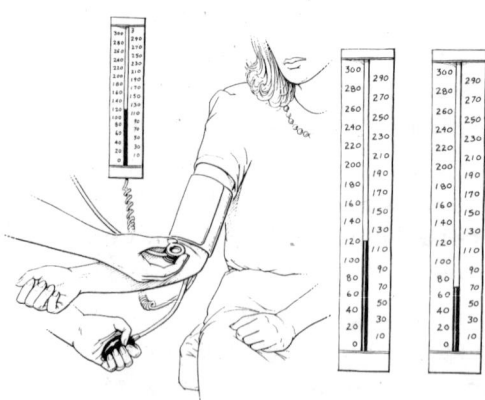

The reading on a mercury column or pressure gauge when the sound of your heartbeat is first heard indicates your systolic pressure. The pressure level on the column or gauge when the sound of your heartbeat can no longer be heard is your diastolic pres-

> **A false reading**
>
> Sometimes a blood pressure measurement can produce false readings that are too high. This happens most often among older adults with damaged arteries that have become very stiff. Although many people with stiff arteries have increased blood pressure, it may not be as high as measurements indicate.
>
> The false readings occur because rigid arteries are difficult to collapse. When a blood pressure measurement is taken, the cuff may not be able to collapse your arm's main (brachial) artery until the cuff's been inflated to a level well above your systolic pressure. And when pressure in the cuff is released, the stiffness causes the artery to open again more quickly than it normally should. Therefore, a blood pressure reading doesn't reflect the true pressure inside your arteries.
>
> Your doctor often can tell whether you have this condition, called pseudohypertension, by feeling your lower arm. Normally, when a blood pressure cuff collapses your brachial artery, the arteries in your lower arm, below the cuff, also collapse so you can't feel them. But among people with very stiff arteries, vessels in their lower arm remain open and can be felt even when no blood is flowing through them.
>
> To get an accurate blood pressure measurement, you may need to have the pressure in your arteries measured by inserting a needle into an artery in your arm.

Receiving a diagnosis

A blood pressure measurement of 140/90 mm Hg is considered high. But one reading of 140/90 mm Hg or higher isn't enough to diagnosis you as having high blood pressure. About 35 percent of people who have high blood pressure on a single reading don't have high blood pressure when their blood pressure is measured again. Only if the reading is extremely high—a systolic pressure of 210 mm Hg or higher or a diastolic pressure of 120 mm Hg or higher—is a diagnosis made based on just one measurement.

Generally, a diagnosis of high blood pressure is made only after at least three visits to your doctor. Your blood pressure is measured two or more times at each visit, for a total of at least six measurements. If the measurements persistently show your blood pressure to be 140/90 mm Hg or higher, then you have high blood pressure.

If you're older than 65 years, your doctor may take even more measurements before deciding you have high blood pressure, because as you get older variations in your blood pressure tend to broaden.

To ensure an accurate reading, it's a good idea not to smoke, eat a big meal or drink caffeine or alcohol for at least 30 minutes before having your blood pressure measured. These factors can all temporarily increase your blood pressure. Also give yourself plenty of time to make it to your appointment. Rushing to an appointment or searching frantically for a parking spot can cause stress, which also can increase your blood pressure temporarily. Before you have your blood pressure measured, sit quietly for a few minutes and try to relax.

And when having your blood pressure taken, don't talk. Talking makes it harder for the person taking your blood pressure to hear the sound of your heartbeat.

Getting an evaluation

Between the time you first learn your blood pressure is high and a diagnosis of high blood pressure is made, your doctor will want to get your medical history, do a physical examination and have you take a few tests.

These three components can provide answers to important questions regarding your treatment and your risk for future health problems, such as:
- Has your high blood pressure damaged any of your organs?
- Is your high blood pressure essential or secondary? Although secondary high blood pressure is uncommon, it's important that each person with high blood pressure be considered for secondary causes of the disease.
- Do you have other risk factors that put you at increased risk for a heart attack or stroke, such as tobacco use, obesity, an inactive lifestyle, high blood cholesterol or diabetes?

If it's unclear whether you have high blood pressure, these evaluation steps can also help confirm the diagnosis.

Medical history

Your medical history may point to a certain factor or event that triggered the increase in your blood pressure. Information from your history also can help your doctor assess your risk for other health conditions.

Do you have "white-coat" hypertension?

Some people—knowingly or unknowingly—become anxious when they have their blood pressure measured. These people may have normal blood pressure at other times, but when it's measured in a medical setting, it's always high. This condition, called "white-coat" hypertension, is fairly common.

If your doctor suspects your high blood pressure is white-coat hypertension, you may need to measure your blood pressure at home and keep a log of your readings. Or, your doctor may recommend that you wear a portable device (ambulatory monitor) that measures your blood pressure periodically throughout the day while you go about your regular activities. These two methods generally give a more realistic and accurate assessment of your blood pressure.

Automated machines in stores and shopping malls that measure blood pressure aren't recommended. These machines are usually accurate when first installed, but they can lose their accuracy if they aren't calibrated often or they're misused.

An important question regarding white-coat hypertension is whether the increase in blood pressure is confined to medical appointments or whether it occurs whenever you feel anxious or stressed. So far, most studies have found the condition to be limited mainly to medical settings. People with white-coat hypertension typically respond to other stress in the same manner as people with normal blood pressure.

White-coat hypertension generally doesn't require drug treatment. However, your doctor may recommend that you adjust your lifestyle to control your weight, get regular physical activity and eat healthfully. You also should see your doctor periodically to monitor for changes in your blood pressure or health that might signal progression from white-coat hypertension to persistent high blood pressure.

During an evaluation, be prepared to answer questions regarding:
- Prior blood pressure readings
- A history of heart or kidney problems, high cholesterol, diabetes or restless sleep or daytime sleepiness due to sleep apnea
- A family history of high blood pressure, heart attack, stroke, kidney disease, diabetes, high cholesterol or early (premature) death

restless sleep or daytime sleepiness due to sleep apnea
- A family history of high blood pressure, heart attack, stroke, kidney disease, diabetes, high cholesterol or early (premature) death
- Symptoms suggesting secondary high blood pressure, such as flushing spells, a rapid heart rate, intolerance to heat or unexplained weight loss
- Alcohol use
- Tobacco use
- Changes in your weight
- Your activity level
- Your diet and use of salt (sodium)

Round-the-clock reading

High blood pressure can, at times, be difficult to diagnose. If your doctor is uncertain you have high blood pressure, or is having trouble determining how severe your condition is, you may need to wear an ambulatory monitor.

The procedure involves fitting you with a portable blood pressure device that you wear for a day. It includes a cuff that fits around your arm and a small monitoring unit that attaches to your belt or clothing. Thin tubes connect the monitor to the cuff. These tubes may be secured to your skin with tape to prevent them from disconnecting.

The monitor is programmed to take your blood pressure about every 10 to 30 minutes over 6 to 24 hours. The device is fully automatic. It pumps up the blood pressure cuff, deflates it and stores the reading in its memory.

You may be a candidate for ambulatory monitoring if you have white-coat hypertension or, just the opposite, you show complications of high blood pressure but have normal blood pressure during medical checkups. Ambulatory monitoring also can be helpful if your blood pressure fluctuates widely or if you're not responding to blood pressure medications.

Keeping a journal that lists your daily activities, the time you did them and any periods of stress, strong emotion or pain also can be helpful. By matching the journal entries with your blood pressure readings, your doctor can see whether certain events or lifestyle factors may be linked to changes in your blood pressure.

Be sure to tell your doctor about *all* the drugs you take—both prescription and over-the-counter, as well as illicit drugs and alternative products, such as herbal and nutritional supplements.

Several prescription and over-the-counter drugs, including many diet pills, decongestant nose sprays and cold, allergy and sinus medicines, can increase your blood pressure. Cocaine and amphetamines also increase blood pressure. In addition, because many alternative products haven't been fully studied to determine their health effects, it's important that you tell your doctor if you're taking such a product—just in case it may be increasing your blood pressure.

Keeping your doctor aware of all the drugs you take can also prevent dangerous interactions should you need to take a blood pressure medication. Some high blood pressure medications don't react well with other drugs. Drug interactions are discussed further in Chapter 12 (page 159).

Physical examination

During the physical examination, your doctor is looking for signs of organ damage. He or she also is checking for abnormalities that might signal a possible cause for the increase in your blood pressure.

Conditions your doctor may check for include:

Narrowed or leaky blood vessels in your eyes. Damage to blood vessels in your eyes is a good indication that blood vessels elsewhere in your body also are damaged.

Heart abnormalities. A fast heart rate, an enlarged heart, an abnormal rhythm or a click or murmur can signal possible heart disease.

Turbulent blood flow. When a blood vessel narrows, it can cause turbulent blood flow that can be heard through a stethoscope. The turbulent flow, called a bruit (BREW-ee), most often occurs in the carotid arteries in your neck and major arteries in your abdomen.

Enlarged kidneys or thyroid gland. These are indications that your high blood pressure may be resulting from another condition.

An aortic aneurysm. It may be felt during examination of your abdomen. A stethoscope also may pick up the sound of blood pulsing through the weakened and bulging blood vessel.

A weakened pulse. A weak pulse in your groin, lower legs and ankles can signal artery damage.

Reduced blood pressure in your ankles. This can result from narrowed or diseased blood vessels in your legs.

Swelling. Accumulation of fluid in your lower legs and ankles is a common symptom of heart or kidney failure.

A decrease in blood pressure when you stand. It can help identify if you may be at risk for fainting or dizziness upon standing (postural hypotension), a side effect of some blood pressure medications.

Routine tests

These tests are commonly part of an evaluation for high blood pressure:

Urinalysis. The presence of protein or red blood cells in your urine can indicate kidney damage. A form of protein in your urine, called microalbuminuria (MI-kroh-al-bu-min-U-ree-ah), can also signal early-stage kidney disease.

In addition, your urine may be tested for the presence of sugar (glucose) resulting from diabetes. Diabetes can make high blood pressure more difficult to control.

Blood chemistry. The amount of sodium and potassium in your blood is measured. Your blood also is tested for levels of certain chemicals, such as creatinine (kree-AT-in-nin), that can indicate damage to your kidneys.

Other common blood tests include measurement of cholesterol-containing blood fats (lipid profile). The higher your total blood cholesterol level and the lower your level of high-density lipoprotein (HDL or "good") cholesterol, the greater your risk for cardiovascular disease. The amount of glucose in your blood also is measured to check for diabetes.

Complete blood cell count. This test determines whether you have an abnormal white or red blood cell count. Its main purpose is to ensure that you don't have other health conditions you may not be aware of, such as a low red blood cell count, called anemia (ah-NEE-me-ah).

Electrocardiogram. Your heart's electrical activity is recorded to check for abnormalities in its rhythm or indications of heart enlargement, heart damage or an inadequate supply of blood to your heart muscle.

Changes in your electrocardiogram (ECG) also can indicate high or low levels of potassium.

Additional tests

If your physical examination and laboratory findings are normal, you probably won't have to have any additional tests. However, further tests may be necessary if you have:
- Sudden onset of high blood pressure or a sharp increase in your usual blood pressure
- Very high blood pressure (180 or higher/110 or higher mm Hg)

- A low blood potassium level
- A bruit over an artery
- Evidence of kidney problems
- Evidence of heart problems
- A possible abdominal aortic aneurysm

Depending on your condition, you may need additional blood or urine tests.

If you have narrowed arteries that are interrupting blood flow, these tests can identify the narrowing and its severity:

Ultrasonography. It uses high-frequency sound waves to show blood flow through an artery. Ultrasonography also is often used to identify specific heart and artery abnormalities.

Magnetic resonance angiography (MRA). This procedure uses the energy created by powerful magnets to view artery blood flow.

Angiography. During this procedure, material that's visible on X-rays is injected into your arteries and then X-rays are taken of specific arteries.

If your doctor suspects you may have a shrunken kidney, an abdominal aortic aneurysm or a tumor, such as an adrenal gland tumor, additional tests may include ultrasonography or one of the following:

Computed tomography. CT scans are three-dimensional X-rays.

Magnetic resonance imaging (MRI). It's similar to MRA, but the scan is focused on a different body area or organ.

Nuclear scanning. It involves injecting radioactive material (radioisotopes) into a vein and then taking nuclear images as the material passes through a specific location or organ. Nuclear scans are used to monitor blood flow, determine the size of an organ or see if an organ is functioning normally.

Deciding on treatment

Treatment of high blood pressure varies with each individual. The type of treatment that works for someone else may not for you. How your high blood pressure is treated depends on your blood pressure stage and the results of your medical history, physical examination and laboratory tests.

There are basically two methods for reducing high blood pressure: lifestyle changes and medication. Depending on your health and your risk factors, recommended lifestyle changes may include losing weight, becoming more active, eating more healthfully, reducing sodium, quitting smoking, limiting alcohol and controlling stress.

As for medication, there are many types that affect your blood pressure in different ways. (That's why it's important that you not share high blood pressure pills with anyone. The medication may not be the same type as yours.)

Latest guidelines

The National Heart, Lung, and Blood Institute, a division of the National Institutes of Health, periodically issues a report on the prevention, detection, evaluation and treatment of high blood pressure.

The latest report, issued in November 1997, divides people with high blood pressure into three risk groups—A, B and C — and makes treatment recommendations for each. Risk is determined according to your blood pressure stage, damage to your internal organs, the presence of cardiovascular disease and factors that increase your risk for cardiovascular disease.

The report also includes recommendations for treating borderline (high-normal) blood pressure. If you have high-normal blood pressure and don't bring it back down to a normal level, there's a good chance it will progress to high blood pressure.

Risk Group A. You're in this risk group if you have high-normal blood pressure or high blood pressure but you don't have organ damage, cardiovascular disease or other risk factors for cardiovascular disease, such as tobacco use or high cholesterol.

If your blood pressure is in the high-normal range, recommended treatment is lifestyle changes to reduce your blood pressure to a normal or optimal level.

If you have stage 1 high blood pressure, lifestyle changes are also the recommended approach. But if after a year these changes fail to reduce your blood pressure to a normal or optimal level, then you may need medication.

If you have stage 2 or stage 3 high blood pressure, initial treatment should include medication in addition to changes in your lifestyle.

Risk Group B. Most people with high blood pressure are in this risk group. It includes people who don't have organ damage or cardiovascular disease but who do have one or more cardiovascular risk factors, excluding diabetes.

If your blood pressure is high-normal, lifestyle changes are recommended.
If you have stage 1 high blood pressure, lifestyle changes are the first

Guidelines for treatment

Blood pressure stages (mm Hg)	Risk Group A	Risk Group B	Risk Group C
High-normal (130-139/85-89)	Lifestyle changes	Lifestyle changes	Medication* Lifestyle changes
Stage 1 (140-159/90-99)	Lifestyle changes (up to 12 months)	Lifestyle changes† (up to 6 months)	Medication Lifestyle changes
Stages 2 and 3 (≥160/≥100)	Medication Lifestyle changes	Medication Lifestyle changes	Medication Lifestyle changes

*For people with heart failure, kidney failure or diabetes.
†If you have multiple risk factors, your doctor may consider drugs as initial therapy plus lifestyle modification.

Major risk factors that can affect treatment

Tobacco use
Undesirable blood fat (lipid) levels
Diabetes
Older than 60 years
A man or postmenopausal woman
Family history of cardiovascular disease

Organ damage or disease that can affect treatment

Heart disease
  Muscle thickening in main pumping chamber
  Previous heart attack or chest pain (angina)
  Prior bypass surgery or angioplasty
  Heart failure
Stroke or transient ischemic attack (mini-stroke)
Kidney disease
Peripheral artery damage
Retinal damage

Modified from National Institutes of Health. The Sixth Report of the Joint National Committee on Prevention, Detection, Evaluation, and Treatment of High Blood Pressure, 1997.

line of treatment. If after 6 months they don't reduce your blood pressure, you may need medication. If you have several risk factors, your doctor may prescribe medication right away, in addition to lifestyle changes.

If you have stage 2 or stage 3 high blood pressure, initial treatment should include both lifestyle changes and medication.

Risk Group C. This group includes people at greatest risk for heart attack, stroke or other problems related to high blood pressure. You fit into this group if you have cardiovascular disease, organ damage, diabetes or a combination of these.

Medication and lifestyle changes are the recommended therapy for all people in this group. Even if your blood pressure is only high-normal, but you have kidney disease, heart failure or diabetes, you should be taking medication.

A common misconception

Many people taking high blood pressure medication believe that it's not important to make changes in their lifestyle because their medication is taking care of their problem. This isn't true.

Sometimes medication can reduce your blood pressure by only a certain amount. And that amount may not be enough to bring your blood pressure down to a normal or optimal level. However, lifestyle changes in addition to your medication often can help you reach a normal pressure.

If your blood pressure is normal, lifestyle changes may help reduce the amount of medication you need daily. Less medication means less cost. In addition, if your medication causes bothersome side effects, cutting back on how much you take may reduce the side effects. A few people who've significantly changed their lifestyle have even been able to stop taking medication entirely, with the help of their doctors.

Finally, lifestyle changes are important for all people with high blood pressure because they can help reduce risk for future health problems, including stroke, heart attack and heart or kidney failure.

Becoming an active partner

It takes a team effort to treat high blood pressure successfully. Your doctor can't do it alone, and neither can you. The two of you need to work together to bring your blood pressure down to a safe level—and keep it there.

However, even though it's a team effort, you can assume most of the responsibility for controlling your blood pressure. Changing your lifestyle—losing weight, becoming more active and eating more healthfully—is an important step within your control. Taking medication regularly and properly is also your responsibility.

Numbers not keeping pace

Since 1972, when the National Heart, Lung, and Blood Institute began an intensive education campaign, there's been steady improvement in awareness, treatment and control of high blood pressure. In return, death and disability attributed to the disease have declined significantly. Death rates from stroke have dropped by nearly 60 percent, and deaths due to heart attack have declined by more than 50 percent.

But during the '90s, these dramatic improvements have slowed and some of the increases have even begun to reverse. Latest results from the National Health and Nutrition Examination Survey (NHANES) show a small decline in all three categories—high blood pressure awareness, treatment and control.

	NHANES II, 1976-80	NHANES III (phase 1), 1988-91	NHANES III (phase 2), 1991-94
Awareness	51%	73%	68.4%
Treatment	31%	55%	53.6%
Control*	10%	29%	27.4%

*Systolic pressure less than 140 mm Hg and diastolic pressure less than 90 mm Hg.
Note: Data are for adults ages 18 to 74 years with systolic pressure of 140 mm Hg or more or diastolic pressure 90 mm Hg or more or taking blood pressure medication.
From National Institutes of Health. The Sixth Report of the Joint National Committee on Prevention, Detection, Evaluation, and Treatment of High Blood Pressure, 1997.

The reason for this overall decline is uncertain. An increase in obesity among Americans is believed to be one factor. Another may be complacency. Above-normal blood pressures may too often be looked on—by both doctors and their patients—as being "close enough."

Remember, you can live a long and healthy life with high blood pressure. But to do that, you need to recognize high blood pressure as a serious condition and become actively involved in its treatment.

Wrap-up

Key points to remember from this chapter:
- A diagnosis of high blood pressure generally is made after three separate doctor visits that show persistently high systolic or diastolic pressure, or both.
- Routine tests, a physical examination and a medical history are typically part of the process to diagnose high blood pressure.
- Appropriate treatment of high blood pressure depends on blood pressure stage, organ damage, cardiovascular risk factors and other diseases.
- The two methods for lowering blood pressure are lifestyle changes and medication.
- Even if you take medication, changes in your lifestyle are essential to controlling high blood pressure.
- Awareness, treatment and control of high blood pressure in the United States have declined slightly in recent years.

Chapter 4

Controlling Your Weight

Your weight and your blood pressure are closely related. When your weight increases, your blood pressure often does too. Considering that Americans are becoming increasingly obese, it's not surprising that weight has become a major factor in the development of high blood pressure. If you're overweight, your risk for development of high blood pressure is two to six times greater than if your weight were healthy.

Fortunately, just as blood pressure can go up when you gain weight, it usually goes down when you lose weight. One of the best ways to reduce high blood pressure is to lose weight. Even shedding a few pounds can bring noticeable blood pressure benefits.

Various programs, formulas and diet plans offer to help you lose weight. However, the most successful method for losing weight—and keeping it off—is to change your eating and activity habits and slim down slowly.

Weight and blood pressure

Being overweight doesn't guarantee that you'll have high blood pressure—you can be overweight and still have normal blood pressure—but it significantly increases your chances.

A 1998 study involving more than 82,000 women found that women who gained 11 to 22 pounds (5 to 10 kilograms) during adulthood had a

70 percent increase in risk for high blood pressure compared with women who didn't gain weight after age 18. For women who gained more than 22 pounds (10 kilograms), their risk was even higher. Although the study didn't include men, other studies involving men also have found that being overweight increases risk for high blood pressure.

What's the link? As you put on weight, you gain mostly fatty tissue. Just like other parts of your body, this tissue relies on oxygen and nutrients in your blood to survive. As demand for oxygen and nutrients increases, the amount of blood circulating through your body also increases. More blood traveling through your arteries means added pressure on your artery walls.

Another reason blood pressure commonly increases among people who are overweight is that weight gain typically increases the level of insulin in blood. This increase in insulin is associated with retention of sodium and water, which increases blood volume.

In addition, excess weight often is associated with an increase in your heart rate and a reduction in the capacity of your blood vessels to transport blood. These two factors also can increase blood pressure.

However, there is good news. The same study that found being overweight increases high blood pressure risk also found that losing weight decreases your risk for high blood pressure. Overweight women who lost 11 to 22 pounds (5 to 10 kilograms) lowered their risk by 15 percent. And women who lost more than 22 pounds (10 kilograms) cut their risk by more than 25 percent.

If you already have high blood pressure, losing weight can help prevent the need for medication. If you're already taking medication, weight loss can help control your blood pressure and possibly reduce how much medication you need each day—perhaps even eliminate your need for medication. However, even though you may no longer be taking medication, you're still at risk for high blood pressure returning. Therefore, you need to monitor your blood pressure regularly.

Overweight vs. obesity

The difference between being overweight and obese is a matter of degree. Federal guidelines define overweight as having a body mass index (BMI) of 25 to 29. Obesity refers to a BMI of 30 or more.

Body mass index is a formula that considers your weight and your

> **Just a little means a lot**
>
> You don't have to lose a large amount of weight to lower your blood pressure. Losing as little as 10 pounds (4.5 kilograms) may be enough to reduce your blood pressure from borderline (high-normal) to normal, or from stage 1 to high-normal.
>
> Shedding just a few pounds also can improve your cholesterol level and reduce your risk for heart attack, stroke and diabetes.
>
> If you're overweight, reducing your weight by 10 pounds may be a good goal. Once you've achieved that goal, you can try for another 10 if you need to lose more. Over a few years—depending on how much weight you need to lose—those 10-pound losses can add up to a significant improvement in your weight and health.

height in determining whether you have a healthful or unhealthful percentage of total body fat. It's a better measurement of health risks related to your weight than using your bathroom scale or standard weight-and-height tables. Unlike weight-and-height tables, body mass index doesn't differentiate between men and women.

To determine your body mass index, locate your height on the chart on the next page and follow it across until you reach the weight nearest to yours. Look at the top of the column for the BMI rating. (If your weight is less than the weight nearest to yours, your BMI may be slightly less. If your weight is greater than the weight nearest to yours, your BMI may be slightly greater.) A BMI of 19 to 24 is considered healthy. A BMI of 25 to 29 signifies overweight, and a BMI of 30 or more indicates obesity.

According to federal guidelines, more than 50 percent of American adults are overweight or obese—almost a third of adults are overweight and nearly another quarter are obese. In almost 40 years, the percentage of overweight Americans has increased only slightly, but the percentage of people who are obese has almost doubled.

Typically, the more you weigh, the greater your risk for health problems. Obesity significantly increases your risk for diabetes, heart disease, stroke and some cancers—in addition to high blood pressure.

What's your BMI?

Body mass index (BMI)

BMI	Healthy		Overweight					Obesity			
	19	24	25	26	27	28	29	30	35	40	45	50
Height	Weight in pounds										
4'10"	91	115	119	124	129	134	138	143	167	191	215	239
4'11"	94	119	124	128	133	138	143	148	173	198	222	247
5'0"	97	123	128	133	138	143	148	153	179	204	230	255
5'1"	100	127	132	137	143	148	153	158	185	211	238	264
5'2"	104	131	136	142	147	153	158	164	191	218	246	273
5'3"	107	135	141	146	152	158	163	169	197	225	254	282
5'4"	110	140	145	151	157	163	169	174	204	232	262	291
5'5"	114	144	150	156	162	168	174	180	210	240	270	300
5'6"	118	148	155	161	167	173	179	186	216	247	278	309
5'7"	121	153	159	166	172	178	185	191	223	255	287	319
5'8"	125	158	164	171	177	184	190	197	230	262	295	328
5'9"	128	162	169	176	182	189	196	203	236	270	304	338
5'10"	132	167	174	181	188	195	202	209	243	278	313	348
5'11"	136	172	179	186	193	200	208	215	250	286	322	358
6'0"	140	177	184	191	199	206	213	221	258	294	331	368
6'1"	144	182	189	197	204	212	219	227	265	302	340	378
6'2"	148	186	194	202	210	218	225	233	272	311	350	389
6'3"	152	192	200	208	216	224	232	240	279	319	359	399
6'4"	156	197	205	213	221	230	238	246	287	328	369	410

Modified from National Institutes of Health Clinical Guidelines on the Identification, Evaluation, and Treatment of Overweight and Obesity in Adults, 1998.

Finding your healthy weight

What is a healthy weight? If you have high blood pressure, or if you're at risk, it's not critical that you become "thin." But you should try to achieve or maintain a weight that improves control of your blood pressure and also lessens your risks for other health problems.

Three do-it-yourself evaluations can tell you whether your weight is healthy or whether you could benefit from losing a few pounds.

Body mass index

The first step in determining your healthy weight is to figure out your body mass index. You can do that by using the accompanying BMI chart.

A BMI of 19 to 24 is desirable. If your BMI is 25 to 29, you're overweight. You're considered obese if you have a BMI of 30 or more. Extreme obesity is a BMI of more than 40.

You're at increased risk for development of a weight-related disease, such as high blood pressure, if your BMI is 25 or greater.

Waist circumference

This measurement is second to your BMI in importance. It indicates where most of your fat is located. People who carry most of their weight around their waists are often referred to as "apples." Those who carry most of their weight below their waist, around their hips and thighs, are known as "pears."

Generally, it's better to have a pear shape than an apple shape. Fat accumulation around your waist is associated with an increased risk for high blood pressure, in addition to other diseases such as diabetes, coronary artery disease, stroke and certain types of cancer. That's because fat in your abdomen is more likely to break down and accumulate in your arteries, although the exact mechanism for how this occurs hasn't been proven.

To determine whether you're carrying too much weight around your abdomen, measure your waist circumference. Find the highest point on each of your hip bones and measure across your abdomen just above those highest points. A measurement of more than 40 inches (102 centimeters) in men and 35 inches (88 centimeters) in women signifies increased health risks, especially if you have a BMI of 25 or more.

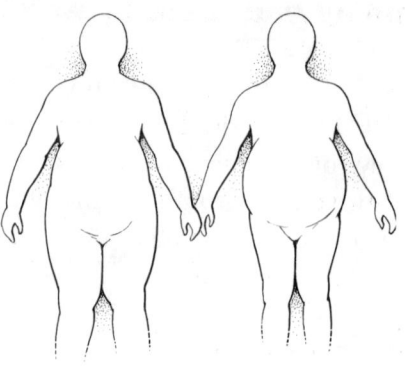

It's not only how much you weigh that's important but also where your body stores extra fat. For two people with the same body mass index, the person with more of an "apple-shape" has a higher risk for health problems than the person who's "pear-

"Pear-shaped"   "Apple-shaped"

Personal and family history

Numbers alone aren't enough. An evaluation of your medical history, along with that of your family, is equally important for determining whether your weight is healthy.

Answer these questions:
- Do you have a health condition, such as high blood pressure, diabetes or high cholesterol, that would benefit from weight loss?
- Do you have a family history of a weight-related illness, such as type 2 diabetes, high blood pressure or sleep apnea?
- Have you gained considerable weight since high school? Weight gain in adulthood is associated with increased health risks.
- Do you smoke cigarettes, have more than two alcoholic drinks per day or live with significant stress? In combination with these behaviors, excess weight can have greater health implications.

Adding up the results

If your BMI shows that you aren't overweight, you're not carrying too much weight around your abdomen and you answered "no" to all of the personal or family history questions, there's probably no health advantage to changing your weight. Your weight is healthy.

If your BMI is between 25 and 29, your waist circumference equals or exceeds healthy guidelines or you answered "yes" to at least one personal and family health question, you may benefit from losing a few pounds. Discuss your weight with your doctor during your next checkup.

If your BMI is 30 or more, clearly, losing some weight will improve your health and reduce your risk for future illness.

Fat factors

Eating too much and exercising too little are most often responsible for weight gain. When you eat more calories than you use during activity, you store excess energy as pounds of fat.

However, overeating and inactivity aren't always the problem. Other factors also can influence your ability to control your weight:

Your genes. Heredity doesn't destine you to be fat, but your genes can make you more susceptible to weight gain. They affect the rate at which your body accumulates fat and where your fat is stored. A family history of obesity increases your chances of becoming obese by about 25 percent to 30 percent.

Other obesity risk factors, such as the foods you eat and your activity habits, are strongly influenced by your family as well.

Your sex. Men can often eat more than women without gaining weight. One explanation is that men have more muscle and muscle uses more energy than fat. Therefore, men use an average of 10 percent to 20 percent more calories than women.

Your age. As you get older, your percentage of muscle tends to drop and fat accounts for a greater percentage of your weight. As a result, your metabolism also slows. Together, these changes reduce your need for calories, often adding an extra pound a year after age 35.

A high-fat, high-calorie diet. You may not overeat, but when you do eat, you consume the wrong things, mainly high-fat or high-calorie foods. Gram for gram, fat provides more than twice as many calories as protein or carbohydrate—9 calories (38 kilojoules) vs. 4 calories (17 kilojoules) per gram.

Many people also mistakenly assume that all foods low in fat are also low in calories. Consuming foods and beverages that are high in calories—even though they may be low in fat—also can result in weight gain.

Medical problems. Less than 5 percent of all cases of obesity can be traced to a health condition, such as a metabolic disorder or a hormonal imbalance. However, some medications, including some oral steroids and antidepressants, commonly result in weight gain.

Steps to successful weight loss

If your BMI is too high and you need to lose weight, here are some steps that can help you lose weight safely and keep it off permanently.

As any veteran dieter knows, losing weight is difficult to do. And it's even more difficult to keep the weight off. Of people who lose weight, most regain it again within 5 years.

There are many products and programs that promise to help you shed pounds. But the best way to reduce your BMI and improve your blood pressure is through lifestyle changes:

Make a commitment. You must be motivated to lose weight because it's what *you* want, not what someone else wants you to do.

Only you can help yourself lose weight. However, that doesn't mean that you have to do everything alone. Your doctor, a registered dietitian or other health care professional can help you develop a plan to lose weight. And don't be afraid to ask for support from your spouse, family and friends.

Think positively. Don't dwell on what you're giving up to lose weight. Instead, concentrate on what you're gaining. Instead of thinking, "I really miss eating a doughnut at breakfast," tell yourself, "I feel a lot better when I eat whole wheat toast and cereal in the morning."

Get your priorities straight. Timing is critical. Don't try to lose weight if you're distracted by other major problems. Chances are, you'll only be setting yourself up for failure.

It takes a lot of mental and physical energy to change habits. If you're having family or financial problems or if you're unhappy with other major aspects of your life, you may be less able to follow through on your good intentions.

Set a realistic goal. Don't try to reach a weight that meets social ideals for thinness and is unrealistic. Instead, try to get to a comfortable weight that you maintained easily as a young adult. Make a healthier lifestyle—not the number of pounds—your primary motivation.

If you've always been overweight, aim for a weight that improves your blood pressure and your blood sugar and blood cholesterol levels. Accept that healthful weight loss is slow and steady. A good weight-loss plan generally involves losing no more than 1 pound (0.5 kilogram) a week if you're a woman and 2 pounds (1 kilogram) a week if you're a man. Men have a higher metabolic rate that speeds weight loss.

Set weekly or monthly goals that allow you to check off your successes.

Know your habits. To become aware of your eating behavior, ask

Commercial weight-loss programs

Many people trying to lose weight find that doing it with others is easier. That's why millions of Americans enroll in commercial weight-loss programs each year. These programs can be helpful, but not all of them approach weight loss in a manner that's safe and effective.

Before you enroll, make sure the program meets the following five criteria:

Safety. The program should ensure that you get adequate nutrition. Although diets may be low in calories, they should still provide the daily recommended amounts of nutrients without the need for unusual supplements or special foods.

Reasonable weight goals. Some people with certain health conditions may benefit from rapid weight loss. But in general, weight loss should be slow and steady. Rapid weight loss is mainly loss of fluid, not fat. Look for a program that's geared toward helping you lose 1 to 2 pounds (0.5 or 1 kilogram) a week. Remember: A loss of just 10 pounds (4.5 kilograms) can have a positive effect on your blood pressure.

Physician participation. The program should encourage consultation with your doctor. Talk with your doctor if you plan to go on a very-low-calorie diet. If you have health problems or you regularly take medication, check with your doctor before taking part in a weight-loss plan.

Attention to permanent lifestyle changes. Losing weight does little good if you can't keep it off. The program also should help you improve your lifelong exercise and eating habits so you can maintain a healthful weight.

Up-front costs. You should know exactly how much the program, including regular follow-up, will cost you.

yourself if you tend to eat when you're bored, angry, tired, anxious, depressed or socially pressured. If you do, try these possible solutions:
- Before eating anything, ask yourself if you really want it.
- Learn to say "no," and stay committed.
- Do something to distract yourself from your desire to eat, such as telephone a friend or run an errand.

- If you're feeling stressed or you're angry, direct that energy constructively. This is a good time for a brisk, 30-minute walk or to clean your closet or the garage.

If you have trouble identifying emotions or situations that cause you to eat, try keeping a notebook. List what, when and why you eat. See if any relationships or patterns emerge.

Change gradually. When you've identified problem behaviors that you'd like to change, remember that gradual changes work best. Choose one area at a time, and be specific about how you're going to improve that behavior. When you've successfully changed one habit, work on another.

Continually practice your new behaviors so they become habits.

Plan ahead. Your old habits may be so ingrained that you do them instinctively. Mentally rehearsing new habits can help. Imagine yourself at a party overflowing with rich hors d'oeuvres or fancy desserts. Envision yourself taking a small portion of a few items and leaving space between them on your plate. Mentally rehearse this plan until you feel you can remember it and do it.

Don't starve yourself. Liquid meals, diet pills and special food combinations aren't your answer to long-term weight control and better health. Four national surveys found that most people try to lose weight by eating 1,000 to 1,500 calories (4,200 to 6,300 kilojoules) a day. However, cutting calories to less than 1,200 (5,040 kilojoules) if you're a woman or 1,400 (5,880 kilojoules) if you're a man doesn't provide enough food to keep you satisfied and you get hungry before your next meal. (See "Calculating your calorie level" to determine your calorie needs.)

Eating fewer than 1,200 calories (5,040 kilojoules) also makes it difficult to get adequate amounts of certain nutrients, such as folic acid, magnesium and zinc. In addition, it promotes temporary loss of fluids and loss of healthy muscle, rather than permanent loss of fat.

Over-the-counter appetite suppressants also aren't recommended if you're trying to lose weight because they contain adrenaline-like substances that can increase your blood pressure.

The best way to lose weight is to eat more healthful foods and change your eating habits. Cutting back on calories from fat allows you to eat more nutrient-rich foods such as whole grains, fruits and vegetables. You also can eat more food for fewer calories. Healthful eating is discussed in more detail in Chapter 6 (page 77).

Get and stay active. Dieting alone will help you lose weight.

But by adding a 30-minute brisk walk most days of the week, you can double your rate of weight loss. Physical activity is the most important factor related to long-term weight loss. It promotes loss of body fat and development of muscle. These changes in body composition help raise the rate at which you burn calories, making it easier to maintain your weight loss.

Aim for at least 30 minutes of moderate activity on most, if not all, days of the week. The next chapter discusses activities that can help you lose weight. Contrary to some people's beliefs, physical activity doesn't have to be strenuous or unenjoyable.

Maintain your progress. Don't let occasional setbacks—and there'll be some—weaken your commitment to lose weight. If you find yourself falling back into an old habit, use the strategies you followed in breaking yourself from that habit in the first place.

Think lifelong. It's not enough to eat healthful foods and exercise for a few weeks or even several months. You have to incorporate these behaviors into your life.

In future years, researchers may uncover more information regarding how genetics and your body contribute to the development of obesity. And, possibly, this information could lead to improved treatments for obesity. However, it's unlikely that these future treatments will ever replace the importance of physical activity and healthful eating in controlling weight.

Calculating your calorie level

Here's an easy way to figure out how many calories you can eat and still lose an average of 1 pound (0.5 kilogram) a week:

_____ x 10 = _____
(current weight in pounds)   (daily calories)

or

_____ x 22 = _____
(current weight in kilograms)   (daily calories)

Use this calorie level as your daily target.

Wrap-up

Key points to remember from this chapter:
- The number of Americans who are overweight or obese continues to increase.
- Your risk for high blood pressure is increased if you've gained more than 10 pounds (4.5 kilograms) as an adult.
- Blood pressure generally increases with weight gain and decreases with weight loss.
- Losing as little as 10 pounds (4.5 kilograms) can lower your blood pressure.
- Aim for a healthful weight, not an ideal one.
- Slow, steady weight loss based on eating healthful foods and getting regular physical activity is the best approach.
- Good weight-loss programs stress safety, a gradual loss of weight and lifestyle changes.

Chapter 5

Getting More Active

One of the most important things you can do to reduce your blood pressure is to become more active. Regular physical activity can lower your blood pressure by about the same amount as many blood pressure medications.

A major reason high blood pressure is so common is that people aren't active enough. Modern conveniences and a shortage of free time have caused Americans to become increasingly sedentary. According to the American Heart Association, only 22 percent of American adults get at least 30 minutes of moderate physical activity most days of the week.

To lower your blood pressure, you don't have to become an athlete. The motto of physical fitness used to be "no pain, no gain." But no more. Moderate activities can be just as beneficial to your blood pressure and overall health, provided you do them regularly. What's important is including more physical activity in your daily routine, not great exhibits of endurance.

Physical activity and blood pressure

Physical activity is critical to controlling your blood pressure because it makes your heart stronger. Your heart is able to pump more blood with less effort. And the less your heart has to work to pump blood, the less force that's exerted on your arteries. In addition, regular activity also helps promote weight loss.

Just how much can regular physical activity reduce your blood pressure? It can lower both your systolic and diastolic pressures by 5 to 10 mm Hg. If you're at risk for high blood pressure, that's enough to keep the condition from developing. If you have high blood pressure, it may be enough to prevent you from having to take medication. If you're taking medication, it's enough to make your medication work more effectively.

In addition to helping control your blood pressure, regular activity also reduces your risk for heart attack, high cholesterol, diabetes, osteoporosis and some cancers. Plus, it:
- Improves concentration
- Promotes more restful sleep
- Reduces fatigue
- Reduces stress and anxiety
- Promotes flexibility and agility (reducing your risk for falls)

Activity vs. intensity

For many years, the common belief was that you had to exercise vigorously if you wanted to become physically fit and improve your health. As a result, people developed an all-or-nothing attitude toward exercise. Unfortunately, too many people were doing nothing.

In 1995, the Centers for Disease Control and Prevention, the American Heart Association, the American College of Sports Medicine and the U.S. Surgeon General issued new guidelines. The guidelines emphasize activity instead of intensity because studies found that less vigorous forms of activity also can improve your health.

"Activity" also became the preferred term over "exercise" because to many people "exercise" implies a planned and repetitive routine. An "activity" doesn't have to be structured to be beneficial.

In addition to common forms of physical activity, such as walking or bicycling, the new guidelines promote activities such as mowing your lawn with a push mower, scrubbing your floors or going dancing. You also can accumulate your activities throughout the day. Ride your bike to the newsstand or spend a few minutes hoeing in your flower bed.

However, not all daily activities count. The activity should be moderately intense. That equates to an effort you perceive as being "fairly light" to "somewhat hard" (see "Perceived Exertion Scale").

The change in emphasis from exercise to activity doesn't eliminate the benefits of vigorous exercise. The new guidelines are meant to complement—not replace—previous advice promoting high-intensity activities. More strenuous activity brings even greater health benefits. The main point is that you take part in some type of physical activity most days of the week.

Perceived Exertion Scale

Moderately intense physical activity qualifies as "fairly light" to "somewhat hard," or about 11 to 14, on the Perceived Exertion Scale. Perceived exertion refers to the total amount of effort, physical stress and fatigue you experience during an activity.

6	
7	Very, very light
8	
9	Very light
10	
11	Fairly light
12	
13	Somewhat hard
14	
15	Hard
16	
17	Very hard
18	
19	Very, very hard
20	

What kind of activity?

Total fitness involves three components—aerobic activity to improve your heart and lung capacity (cardiovascular health), flexibility exercises to improve flexibility in your joints and strengthening exercises to maintain bone and muscle mass.

Of these three, aerobic activity has the greatest effect on controlling your blood pressure. An activity is aerobic if it places added demands on your heart, lungs and muscles, increasing your need for oxygen.

Cleaning house, playing golf or raking leaves are all aerobic activities if they require a fairly light to somewhat hard effort. Other common forms of aerobic activity include:

Walking. Walking is appealing to many people because it doesn't require any special athletic skills or instruction. It's convenient and inexpensive. You can vary your route to keep it interesting. And it's an activity that you can enjoy alone or with friends.

Walking also helps burn calories. You burn about an equal amount of fat during long-duration, low-intensity exercise as you do during short exercise periods.

When walking, make sure you wear good walking shoes that give your feet support and traction. If you've been inactive and are out of shape, begin by walking at a very light pace (see "Perceived Exertion Scale") for 5 to 10 minutes. Each time you walk, gradually increase the intensity and duration.

Jogging. Jogging is an excellent form of aerobic exercise because it works your heart, lungs and muscles in a relatively brief time. This allows many people to fit jogging into their busy schedules. And, like walking, jogging doesn't require a lot of equipment—just a good pair of shoes.

However, jogging requires prior cardiovascular conditioning and muscle strengthening. Over time, jogging also can be damaging to joints in your ankles and knees.

If you'd like to take up jogging but you haven't been active for several months, begin by walking. When you're able to walk 2 miles (1.6 kilometers) in 30 minutes comfortably, you're ready to try alternating jogging with walking. Gradually increase the amount of time you spend jogging and decrease the amount of time you spend walking.

To minimize your risk of injury and muscle and joint discomfort, don't jog more than three or four times a week and try to jog on alternate days.

Bicycling. Like walking, bicycling is a good choice if you're just getting started on a regular exercise program. Start slowly and build up your endurance.

You may be tempted to challenge yourself by setting the gears to make pedaling hard, producing a strain resembling that of a hard run. This doesn't work your heart and lungs effectively, except when you're ascending a hill. Pedaling more rapidly at all times—even while going downhill—will help make your ride an aerobic activity.

Swimming. It's an excellent form of cardiovascular exercise because it conditions your heart, lungs and muscles throughout your body. It's also gentle to your joints. If you have arthritis or another joint disease, swimming is a good way to increase your aerobic activity.

Exercise machines. Exercise machines can build both aerobic capacity and muscular strength. In general, you get what you pay for when you purchase an exercise machine. Look at the warranty—it's usually a sign of quality. Make sure the device is solidly built, with no exposed cables or chains. Avoid spring-operated components, and look for a machine that operates smoothly.

Don't make a purchase decision based on gizmos that monitor your performance. Many of the machines are laden with such things as calorie counters, timers, computer printouts and video displays. They're things you don't need and probably won't use.

Each of these five basic machines offers unique fitness benefits:

Stationary bicycle. It's an excellent choice for both beginning and veteran exercisers. It gives you mainly a lower-body workout, but some bicycles have moving handlebars that also provide an upper-body workout, increasing demands on your heart and lungs. If you have knee problems, be sure the resistance can be adjusted to a low setting, and keep your knees bent throughout the cycle.

Rowing machine. This type of machine offers a good aerobic workout by exercising muscles throughout your body, as well as your heart and lungs. It helps strengthen your back, shoulders, stomach, legs and arms. Machines with a flywheel and chain drive generally are easier to operate and are more effective than piston-type rowers, which are less expensive and more compact. Proper technique is important to avoid back strain.

Treadmill. A treadmill builds leg strength as well as aerobic capacity. Some models offer adjustable inclines that simulate climbing hills. You can adjust the speed for walking or jogging. High horsepower models generally run smoother and are more durable.

Stair-climber. It helps tone and strengthen your hips, buttocks, thighs, hamstrings, calves and lower back. A stair-climber also provides an effective heart and lung workout. Compared with jogging, it reduces wear and tear on your ankles and knees. Still, the device can aggravate existing knee problems.

Cross-country ski machine. Advantages of the machine are that it offers a good overall workout and it's easy on your joints. But some people find it difficult to master. You have to be able to move your arms and legs in rhythmic opposition. This can take practice.

How much activity?

Be as active as you can each day. At a minimum, aim to burn at least 150 calories (630 kilojoules) daily doing aerobic activities. For moderately intense activities, that equals about 30 minutes. Lighter activities require more time, and more vigorous activities less time. In addition, the more you weigh, the less time it takes to burn calories, and the less you weigh, the more time. However, if you use 30 minutes as your guide, you'll be close to getting the minimal amount of activity you need.

If it's difficult to carve 30 minutes out of your busy schedule, you can accumulate your activities in 5- to 10-minute intervals throughout the day. Park your car farther away from work. Take the stairs instead of the elevator. Go for a short walk during your lunch hour. Three 10-minute periods of activity are almost as beneficial to your overall fitness as one 30-minute session.

Also look for opportunities to include more activity within your regular routine. While watching or listening to the news, walk on your tread-

Activity guide

Activity	Minutes required to burn 150 calories in 155-pound person*
Washing and waxing a car	45 to 60
Washing windows and floors	45 to 60
Playing volleyball	45
Playing touch football	30 to 45
Gardening	30 to 45
Wheeling self in wheelchair	30 to 40
Walking (20 minutes per mile)	35
Basketball (shooting baskets)	30
Bicycling (6 minutes per mile)	30
Dancing fast	30
Raking leaves	30
Water aerobics	30
Lawn mowing (push mower)	30
Walking (15 minutes per mile)	30
Swimming laps	20
Basketball (playing a game)	15 to 20
Jogging (12 minutes per mile)	20
Running (10 minutes per mile)	15
Shoveling snow	15
Stairwalking	15

*Equivalent to minutes required to burn 630 kilojoules in 70-kilogram person. Modified from National Institutes of Health Clinical Guidelines on the Identification, Evaluation, and Treatment of Overweight and Obesity in Adults, 1998.

mill. When reading a magazine or book, get on your stationary bicycle.

The 6-step fitness plan that follows spells out more specifically how to start an activity program, how to add time or distance as your fitness improves and how to add strength training to round out your overall fitness.

A 6-step fitness plan

One of the challenges of incorporating more physical activity into your day is just getting out of your chair and doing it. You know that you should be more active, but taking that step from "knowing" to "doing" sometimes isn't as easy as it may seem.

To help you get and stay active, here's a total fitness program that's safe for almost anyone. However, if you have any chronic health conditions or you're at significant risk for cardiovascular disease, some special precautions may apply. To be on the safe side, check with your doctor first if you:

- Have a blood pressure of 160/100 mm Hg or more
- Have cardiovascular or lung disease, diabetes, arthritis or kidney disease
- Are a man age 40 years or older or a woman age 50 or older
- Have a family history of heart-related problems before age 55
- Are unsure of your health status
- Have previously experienced chest discomfort, shortness of breath or dizziness during times when you've exerted yourself

If you take medication regularly, ask your doctor if increasing your physical activity will change how the medication works or its side effects. Drugs for diabetes and cardiovascular disease can sometimes cause dehydration, impaired balance and blurred vision. Some medications can also affect the way your body reacts to exercise.

Step 1: Set your goals

Goals help motivate you to get and stay active. Start with simple goals, such as trying to be active most days of the week, and then progress to longer-range goals. People who can stay physically active for 6 months usually end up making regular activity a habit.

Be sure to set goals you can reasonably achieve. It's easy to get frustrated and give up on goals that are too ambitious. Plus, be specific about your goals. State exactly what your goal is and the time you want to achieve it.

If you have, or are at risk for, high blood pressure, one of your goals should be to lower your blood pressure. Another goal might be to lose weight. Your goals might read as follows:

- I will lower my systolic blood pressure by 4 mm Hg and my diastolic pressure by 2 mm Hg in 6 months.
- I will lose 5 pounds (2.7 kilograms) in 6 months.

To achieve these health goals, it may help you to set some activity goals. These goals should also be attainable and specific. Here are some examples:

- I will stretch before and after physical activity.
- I will walk for 30 minutes 3 days a week.
- I will do strengthening exercises 2 days a week.

Once you've decided on your goals, write them down and keep them where you can see them. Seeing your goals can help motivate you.

As you accomplish your goals, set new ones.

Step 2: Assemble your equipment

Your equipment can be as simple as athletic shoes. Wear shoes that fit your feet well and provide good support.

If you plan to bicycle, make sure your bicycle is adjusted for your height and arm length. When you're seated and have your foot on the pedal nearest the ground, your leg should be not quite fully extended. You also should be able to reach the handlebars and work the brakes and shift mechanism while keeping your eyes on the road.

If you decide to purchase an exercise machine, learn how to adjust it to fit your size and level of endurance.

For strength training, you can make your own weights by filling old socks with beans or pennies, or partially filling a half-gallon milk jug with water or sand. Or you can purchase used weights by the pound at some athletic equipment stores.

Step 3: Take time to stretch

Stretching for 5 to 10 minutes before you begin an activity increases blood flow and limbers up your muscles. This helps prepare your body for your upcoming aerobic activity.

Stretching for 5 to 10 minutes after an aerobic activity—when your muscles are loosened up—improves overall flexibility in your muscles and joints. It also helps prevent muscle soreness and reduces your risk for injury.

Warm-up and cool-down stretches

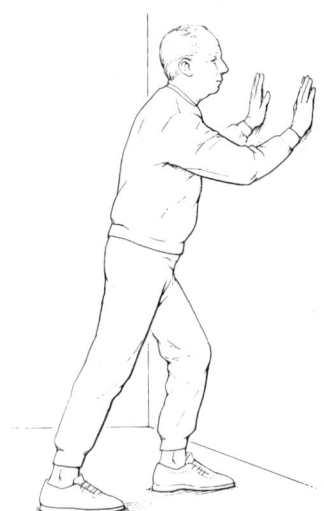

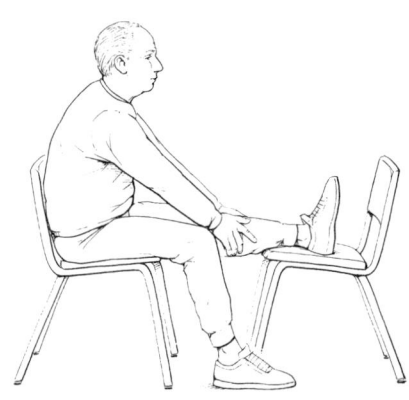

Calf stretch: Stand an arm's length from wall. Lean into wall. Place one leg forward with knee bent. Keep other leg back with knee straight and heel down. Keeping back straight, move hips toward the wall until you feel a stretch. Hold for 30 seconds. Relax. Repeat with the

Hamstring stretch: Sit in a chair with one leg on another chair. Keep back straight. Slowly bend pelvis forward at the hip until you feel a stretch in the back of your thigh. Hold the position for 30 seconds. Relax. Repeat with the other leg. (You also can do this exercise sitting on the floor with one leg out front and the other bent back-

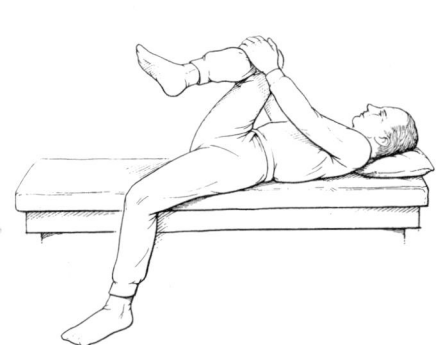

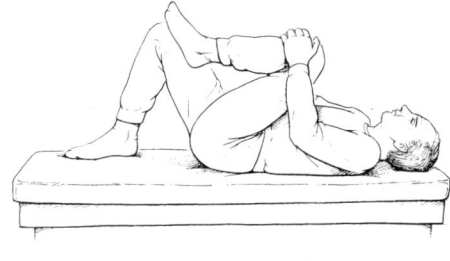

Upper-thigh stretch: Lie on a table or bed with one leg and hip as near the edge as possible and your lower leg hanging relaxed over the edge. Pull your other thigh and knee firmly toward your chest until your lower back flattens against the table. Hold for 30 seconds. Relax. Repeat with the other leg.

Lower-back stretch: Lie on a flat surface, such as the floor or a table, with your hips and knees bent and feet flat on the surface. Pull your left knee toward your shoulder with both hands (if you have knee problems, pull from the back of your thigh). Hold for 30 seconds. Relax. Repeat with the other leg.

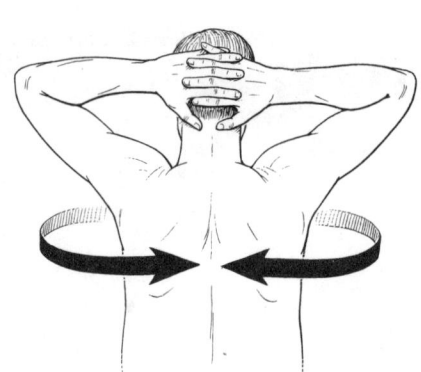

Chest stretch: Clasp your hands behind your head. Pull elbows firmly back while inhaling deeply. Hold for 30 seconds (keep breathing). Relax.

Step 4: Emphasize aerobic fitness

Spend at least 30 minutes doing an aerobic activity you perceive as being fairly light to somewhat hard. If you've been inactive and are out of shape, begin with just 5 to 10 minutes at a very light pace. Then gradually increase your time by 1 to 5 minutes per session and your pace. Many people start with frenzied zeal and then quit when their muscles and joints become sore or injured.

After you've been active for a while and when you feel you're ready, gradually pick up the pace of your activity or increase the time you spend doing it by a few minutes each day. Instead of 30 minutes most days of the week, try aiming for 45 to 60 minutes.

When doing aerobic activities keep these suggestions in mind:

Mix your activities. Doing the same thing all the time increases the chances that you'll become bored and quit being active. Think of activities beyond the common forms, such as canoeing, ballroom dancing or hiking. In addition, try to alternate among activities that emphasize lower- and upper-body fitness.

Participating in a variety of activities also reduces your chance of injury to a specific muscle or overuse of a joint.

Be flexible. If you're overly tired or not feeling well, take a day or two off.

Listen to your body. A few minor aches and pains are bound to occur at times, but be aware of signs of overexertion or stress (see "Avoiding injury," page 75).

> **The talk test**
> One way you can tell whether you're exerting yourself at the right intensity level is if you can carry on a conversation with a companion. If you're too winded to complete a four- to five-word sentence, you're probably pushing too hard and should slow your pace.

Step 5: Build strength

At least twice a week, spend a few minutes doing exercises that help build strength. Greater muscle strength makes aerobic activity easier. A greater percentage of muscle than fat also increases the number of calories you use each day. In addition, stronger muscles, tendons and ligaments around your joints protect you against falls and fractures and reduce your risk for injury.

You build strength by working your muscles against your own body weight, large elastic bands or weighted objects (weights). The amount of weight or resistance you need to build muscle depends on your current strength. Choose a resistance that makes you feel as though you're working at a "somewhat hard" level on the Perceived Exertion Scale.

Simple strengthening exercises

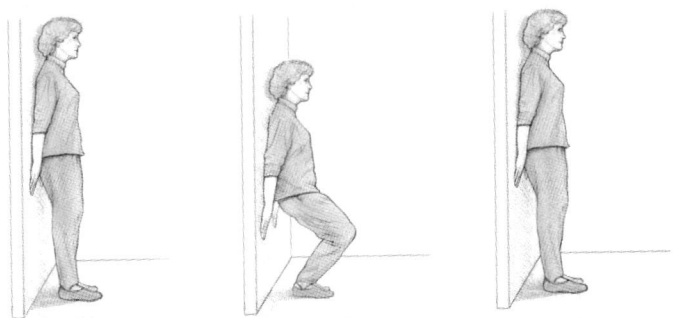

Wall slide: Stand with your heels about 12 inches (30.5 centimeters) from the wall. With your back against the wall, slowly slide down the surface until your knees are bent at a 45-degree angle. Slide back up to a standing position. This strengthens your quadriceps, improving walking and climbing strength.

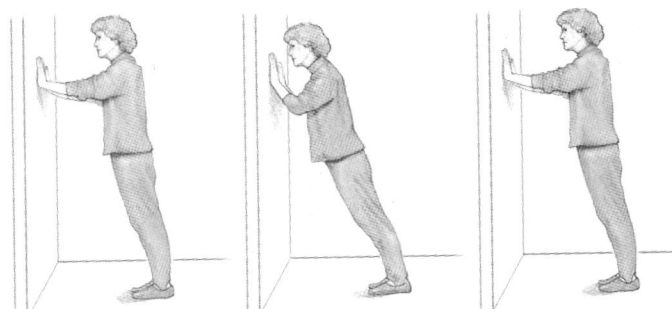

Wall push-up: Face the wall and stand far enough away that you can place your palms on the wall with your elbows slightly bent. Slowly bend your elbows and lean toward the wall, supporting your weight with your arms. Straighten your arms and return to a standing position. This strengthens muscles in your arms and chest.

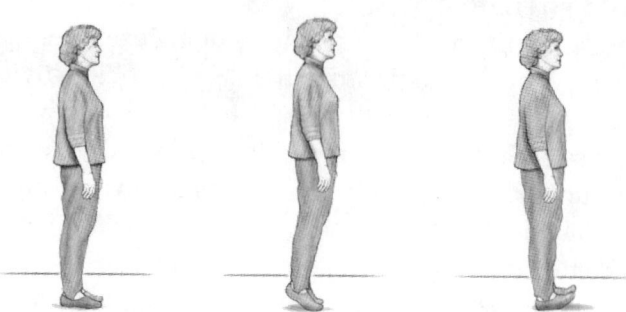

Toe and heel raise: Standing, rise up so your weight is on your toes. Then rock back and shift your weight to your heels, lifting your toes off the ground. This strengthens your calf and lower leg muscles to improve your balance.

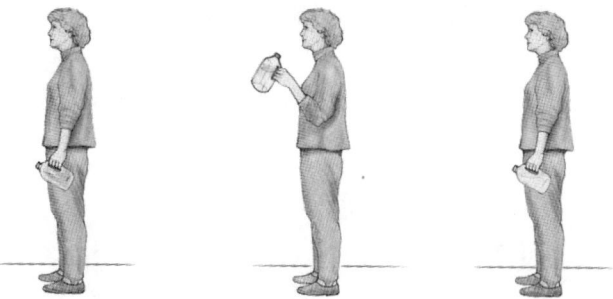

Arm curl: Stand with your feet shoulder-width apart. For resistance, hold a partially filled half-gallon milk jug. Flex your elbow until your hand reaches shoulder height. Hold, then lower your arm slowly. This tones your biceps and helps in carrying and lifting.

At the start, light weights or low resistance and many repetitions help build muscle endurance. As you become stronger, gradually increase the weight or resistance or increase the number of repetitions.

Before doing heavy weight lifting, though, talk to your doctor. The strain of heavy weight lifting can cause a sharp increase in your blood pressure. This could possibly be dangerous if you have uncontrolled high blood pressure.

Step 6: Look for ways to stay motivated

Most people achieve a desirable level of fitness in 3 to 9 months. Your goal then is to maintain your fitness.

To keep up your motivation:

Track your progress. Measure your progress with a written log or diary. Seeing on paper how your fitness has improved can help keep you motivated to do more.

Adapt your activities. As you become more fit, fine-tune the intensity and duration of your activities.

Try new activities. Incorporating different and more challenging activities into your schedule will help keep it enjoyable. Also look for ways to include your family in your physical activities.

Avoiding injury

Injuries do occasionally happen during physical activity. However, you can reduce your risk of an injury by following these tips:

Drink plenty of water. Water helps maintain your normal body temperature and cools working muscles. To help replenish the fluids you lose, drink water before and after your activity.

Dress appropriately. Wear loose-fitting, comfortable clothing that allows perspiration to escape from your body.

Warm up and cool down. Stretching before an aerobic activity prepares your body for the upcoming activity. Stretching afterward helps improve your flexibility.

Be active regularly. Your risk for injury increases if you go back and forth between intense workouts and weeks of inactivity.

Avoid start-and-stop activities. A controlled, continuous form of activity, such as walking or cycling, generally produces less risk for a muscle pull or other injury than activities in which you start and stop frequently, such as basketball or tennis.

Don't compete. Avoid the physical and emotional intensity that often accompanies competitive sports.

Let food digest. Wait 2 to 3 hours after eating a large meal before being active. Digestion directs blood toward your digestive system and away from your heart.

Tailor your activity to the weather. When it's hot and humid, reduce your speed and distance. Or exercise early in the morning or later in the evening when it's cooler.

Avoid activity near heavy traffic. Breathing carbon monoxide given off by automobiles reduces the oxygen supply to your heart.

Know the warning signs. Seek immediate care if you experience any of these:
- Tightness in your chest
- Severe shortness of breath
- Chest pain or pain in your arms or jaw, often on the left side
- Fast, irregular heartbeats (palpitations)
- Dizziness, faintness or feeling sick to your stomach

Moderate activity shouldn't cause discomfort. Your breathing may be increased and you should feel like you're working. However, you shouldn't feel pain or experience exhaustion.

Wrap-up

Key points to remember from this chapter:
- Regular physical activity can reduce your blood pressure by 5 to 10 mm Hg.
- Regular activity is more important than intensity.
- You should get at least 30 minutes of moderately intense activity most, if not all, days of the week. If you've been inactive, gradually work up to this amount.
- Aerobic activity has the greatest effect on blood pressure. An activity is aerobic if it places added demands on your heart, lungs and muscles, increasing your need for oxygen.
- If time is a problem, look for ways to include more activity in your daily routine.
- Include a variety of activities. You're more likely to stay active if you're doing things you enjoy.
- The health benefits of physical activity are almost always much greater than your risk for injury.

Chapter 6

Eating Well

In addition to controlling your weight and becoming more active, eating more healthfully also can help lower your blood pressure and keep it under control. Together, these three steps can lessen the chances you'll need medication.

Eating well doesn't mean counting calories and giving up all of the foods you enjoy. It means enjoying a variety of foods that can keep you healthy now and in the years ahead. A variety of foods helps ensure you get the right mix of nutrients.

For managing high blood pressure, avoiding excessive sodium is still recommended, as discussed in the next chapter. But the newest information suggests that eating less fat and more grains, fruits, vegetables and low-fat dairy products not only promotes your overall health but also has specific benefits for blood pressure control.

The DASH study

Over the years, several studies have suggested that a healthful diet can reduce your blood pressure. Now there's proof it's true.

A 1997 study called "Dietary Approaches to Stop Hypertension," or DASH, compared three diets among 459 people. The group included people with high blood pressure and those with borderline (high-normal) blood pressure at risk for development of high blood pressure.

Of the three diets in the study, one matched the typical American diet. It was low in fruits, vegetables and dairy products and had a fat content typical of the average American diet (37 percent of total calories). Another diet stressed fruits and vegetables—a minimum of 8 servings—but it didn't control intake of dairy products or fat. The third diet, called the combination diet, stressed fruits and vegetables plus ample grains and low-fat dairy products. Fat was also lower than that of the other diets (less than 30 percent of total calories).

The result: Both the fruit-and-vegetable diet and the combination diet lowered blood pressure. But the combination diet produced the greatest reductions in blood pressure.

People with high blood pressure on the combination diet experienced an average decrease of 11.4 mm Hg in systolic pressure and 5.5 mm Hg in diastolic pressure. That's about the same effect as some medications. People with high-normal blood pressure reduced their systolic pressure an average of 3.5 mm Hg and their diastolic pressure an average of 2 mm Hg.

Researchers aren't certain why the combination diet fared better. But they believe it may be because the diet promotes weight loss and because it's rich in potassium, calcium and magnesium, minerals linked with lower blood pressure.

Sodium in all three diets was limited to about 3,000 milligrams (mg) daily—less than what most Americans typically consume. A follow-up DASH study is examining whether lowering sodium further can result in even greater reductions in blood pressure.

Basic principles of DASH

The DASH eating plan is rich in grains, fruits, vegetables and low-fat dairy products. By emphasizing these foods, the plan limits fat, saturated fat and cholesterol, while providing plentiful amounts of fiber, potassium, calcium and magnesium.

Although research suggests that the DASH diet may specifically help lower high blood pressure, the premise of the diet is similar to the Food Guide Pyramid, recommended for all healthy Americans. Both plans promote eating more grains, fruits and vegetables and fewer animal products, including meat, poultry and fish.

The DASH plan, however, recommends a minimum of 8 servings of fruits and vegetables instead of the 5 suggested in the Food Guide

Pyramid. The DASH plan also separates vegetable from animal proteins, recommending 4 to 5 servings a week of nuts, seeds and legumes. In this way, the DASH diet further limits fat and helps ensure more fiber, plus potassium and magnesium, nutrients associated with lower blood pressure.

How to eat with DASH

To manage your blood pressure with your diet, here are the types and amounts of foods to eat every day:

Grains: 7 to 8 servings. Grains include breads, cereals, rice and pasta. In addition to being low in fat, grains are rich in complex carbohydrates and nutrients. Whole grains provide more fiber and nutrients, such as magnesium, than refined varieties.

Breads and pasta are naturally low in fat and calories. To keep them that way, be selective about what you add to these foods. Avoid cream and cheese sauces on pasta and choose instead vegetable or fresh tomato-based toppings.

Select plain yeast breads rather than quick breads, sweet rolls or other baked goods with added fat.

Fruits and vegetables: 8 to 10 servings. Eating more fruits and vegetables may be one of the best things you can do to improve your blood pressure and your overall health. In addition to being virtually fat-free and low in calories, fruits and vegetables provide fiber and a variety of nutrients, including potassium and magnesium. They also contain phytochemicals, substances that can reduce your risk of cardiovascular disease and some cancers.

Substituting fruits and vegetables for foods that have more fat and calories is also a relatively easy way to improve your diet without cutting back on the amount you eat. The key is not to smother your fruits and vegetables with dips or sauces that contain a lot of fat.

Dairy products: 2 to 3 servings. Dairy products are key sources of calcium and vitamin D, which helps your body absorb calcium. They also provide protein. But dairy products can be high in fat. By choosing low-fat or fat-free varieties, such as skim or low-fat milk and yogurt, and fat-free or part-skim cheeses, you can get the health benefits of dairy products without all the fat.

Meat, poultry and fish: 2 or fewer servings. These foods are rich sources of protein, B vitamins, iron and zinc. When you do eat meat, choose lean cuts, such as tenderloin, round or sirloin. When preparing poultry, remove the skin to reduce fat by about half. However, because even lean varieties contain fat and cholesterol, try to limit all animal foods.

Fish is one of the leanest animal proteins you can choose. In addition, the fat it does contain is mainly a type called omega-3 fatty acids.

The DASH diet

This is the plan that reduced blood pressure by the greatest amount in the DASH study. To help control your blood pressure, try to eat daily the amounts listed from the different food groups.

Food & daily servings	Serving examples
Grains 7 to 8	½ cup (3 oz./90 g) cooked cereal, rice or pasta ½ cup (1 oz./30 g) ready-to-eat cereal ½ slice whole-wheat (wholemeal) sandwich bread ½ bagel or English muffin
Fruits & vegetables 8 to 10	¼ cup (1½ oz./45 g) raisins ¾ cup (6 fl. oz./180 mL) 100% fruit juice 1 medium apple or banana 12 grapes 1 cup (2 oz./60 g) raw leafy green vegetables ½ cup (3 oz./90 g) cooked vegetables 1 medium potato
Dairy products 2 to 3	1 cup (8 fl. oz./250 mL) low-fat or fat-free milk or 1 cup (8 oz./250 g) yogurt 1½ oz. (45 g) reduced-fat or fat-free cheese 2 cups (16 oz./500 g) low-fat or fat-free cottage cheese
Meat, poultry & fish 2 or fewer	2-3 oz. (60-90 g) cooked skinless poultry, seafood or lean meat
Legumes, nuts & seeds 4 to 5 a week	½ cup (3½ oz./105 g) cooked legumes ¼ cup (1 oz./30 g) seeds ⅓ cup (1 oz./30 g) nuts

Serving amounts are based on a diet of 2,000 calories (8,400 kilojoules) per day. Most Americans need between 1,600 and 2,400 calories (6,700 to 10,080 kilojoules) daily, depending on age and activity. To adjust the diet to include fewer or more servings, talk to a registered dietitian.

Modified from National Institutes of Health. The DASH Diet.

Omega-3s may help lower your blood pressure slightly, and they help thin your blood and reduce your risk of clots. Blood clots that form in narrowed arteries increase your risk of heart attack and stroke.

Legumes, nuts and seeds: 4 to 5 servings a week. Legumes include beans, dried peas and lentils, which are low in fat and have no cholesterol. They're an excellent source of plant protein. Legumes, nuts and seeds provide a variety of nutrients, including magnesium and potassium, plus phytochemicals and fiber.

Although nuts and seeds contain fat, most of it is monounsaturated, the type that may help protect against coronary artery disease.

Menus with DASH

To help you get started on a more healthful diet, see the menus and recipes in the back of the book that incorporate the DASH eating plan. They begin on page 167.

Do you eat enough fruits and vegetables?

If you're like most people, you don't. Yet, getting 8 to 10 servings daily is easier than you may think.

Here are several suggestions for adding more fruits and vegetables into your day:
- Have a glass of 100 percent fruit or vegetable juice for breakfast.
- Top your morning cereal with blueberries, raspberries or a sliced banana.
- Eat a small salad with your lunch or dinner.
- Add tomatoes, sprouts or greens to your sandwich.
- Have a bowl of vegetable soup.
- Snack on a piece of fruit or raw vegetables.
- Add vegetables to your casseroles.
- Top your baked potato with cooked broccoli, cauliflower and carrots.
- Substitute spinach, summer squash or eggplant for meat with your pasta.
- Have berries with your yogurt or use them as topping on desserts.

A closer look at three important minerals

The DASH diet emphasizes the benefits of three minerals—potassium, calcium and magnesium—that are key factors in managing high blood pressure. This table summarizes the effects of the minerals on blood pressure and what foods contain them.

Mineral	How it works	Where it is
Potassium	Balances the amount of sodium in your cells	Many fruits and vegetables, whole grains, legumes, dairy products
Calcium	Not proven to prevent high blood pressure, but too little is linked with higher blood pressure	Dairy products, green leafy vegetables, fish with edible bones, calcium-fortified foods
Magnesium	Too little is linked with higher blood pressure	Legumes, green leafy vegetables, nuts and seeds, whole grains

Good sources of potassium

These foods have moderate to very high amounts of potassium in each serving. (For serving sizes, see table on page 80.) You'll find that some foods are listed more than once, due to how they're prepared or preserved.

	Fruits	Vegetables	Other
Moderate	Apple, raw or juice Blackberries Cherries, sour, canned Grape juice Grapefruit Grapefruit juice Grapes Mandarin orange Peaches, canned or fresh Pear, fresh Pineapple, canned, fresh or juice Plums, canned or fresh	Asparagus Broccoflower Broccoli Cabbage Carrots, canned or raw Corn Eggplant Green beans Kale Lettuce Mixed vegetables, frozen Parsley Peas	

Good sources of potassium (continued)

	Fruits	Vegetables	Other
	Raisins Raspberries	Rhubarb, fresh or frozen Turnips	
High	Apricots, whole and dried Banana Cherries, sweet red Dates Figs, raw, dried Guava Kiwifruit Mango Nectarine Orange Orange juice Passion fruit juice Prune juice Prunes Strawberries Tangerines Watermelon	Artichoke Bamboo shoots Beans, dried Beets Broccoli Brussels sprouts Collards, cooked Kohlrabi, cooked Mixed vegetables, canned Mushrooms Okra Parsnips, cooked Potatoes, mashed, pieces or plain chips Pumpkin Rutabaga, cooked Spinach Squash Sweet potatoes, canned Tomato, canned whole or spaghetti sauce Tomato juice Vegetable juice cocktail Wax beans, canned Zucchini	Cocoa mixes, 1/4 cup (1 oz./30 g) powder Milk, 1 cup (8 fl. oz./250 mL) Peanut butter, 2 tbsp. Yogurt, 1 cup (8 oz./250 g)
Very high	Cantaloupe Elderberries Honeydew Papaya	Avocado Bamboo shoots, raw Carrot juice Chicory Potato, baked Sweet potato, baked Swiss chard, boiled Water chestnuts, fresh	Chocolate milk, 1 cup (8 fl. oz./250 mL) Potassium chloride salt substitutes, 1/4 tsp. Potato chips, flavored (1 oz./30 g)

What about supplements?

A healthful diet should provide adequate potassium, calcium and magnesium. Getting these nutrients from foods instead of supplements helps ensure the right mix of nutrients only food can provide.

If you're taking a diuretic (DI-u-RET-ik) medication that causes your body to lose potassium, your doctor may recommend a potassium supplement if your diet isn't providing enough.

Calcium and magnesium supplements generally aren't necessary to control high blood pressure.

Your 15 best sources of calcium

It's recommended that adults get between 1,000 and 1,200 milligrams of calcium daily. Here are the foods that can help you reach that amount.

	Calcium (milligrams)
Milk, fat-free and low-fat, 1 cup (8 fl. oz./250 mL)	300
Tofu set with calcium, ½ cup (4 oz./125 g)	258
Yogurt, 1 cup (8 oz./250 g)	250
Orange juice, calcium-fortified, 1 cup (8 fl. oz./250 mL)	240
Ready-to-eat cereal, calcium-fortified, 1 cup (1½ oz./45 g)	200
Mozzarella cheese, part-skim, ¼ cup (1 oz./30 g)	183
Canned salmon with bones (3 oz./90 g)	181
Collard greens, cooked, ½ cup (3 oz./90 g)	179
Ricotta cheese, part-skim, ¼ cup (2 oz./60 g)	169
Bread, calcium-fortified, 2 slices	160
Cottage cheese, low-fat, 1 cup (8 oz./250 g)	138
Parmesan cheese, 2 tbsp.	138
Navy beans, cooked, 1 cup (7 oz./220 g)	128
Turnips, cooked, ½ cup (3 oz./90 g)	125
Broccoli, cooked, 1 cup (2 oz./60 g)	94

Common sources of magnesium

Magnesium is found in a wide variety of foods and in drinking water.

Regularly eating green leafy vegetables, whole grains, legumes and even small amounts of meat, poultry and fish will ensure you get an adequate amount. Nuts and seeds are also good sources of magnesium.

A fresh approach to shopping

You don't have to drastically change the way you shop to eat well. But some simple strategies can help you shop more wisely and follow the DASH eating plan:

Make a list. Decide on the meals you're going to make during the coming week and include the ingredients you need on your grocery list. Also think of what you'll need for breakfast and snacks. As you start eating more nutritiously, you'll notice more fruits, vegetables, breads and cereals on your list. Foods you may have thought of as side dishes, such as pasta, rice and beans, will also become more prominent on your list.

Buy fresh. Fresh foods are generally better than ready-to-eat foods because you can control what ingredients are added. Plus, fresh foods generally have more flavor and color.

Don't shop on an empty stomach. If you shop when you're hungry, you may be tempted to buy foods you don't need, and these are often high in fat, calories and sodium.

Look at the labels. Take time to read food labels. They can help you compare similar foods and select items that are the most nutritious.

How to use food labels

Since May 1994, packaged goods sold in the United States have carried the Nutrition Facts label. Nutrition Facts are an at-a-glance method for verifying how a food fits into your eating plan.

Each label contains information pertaining to:

Serving size. Look at the serving size and servings per container. See if the serving size is similar to the amount you actually eat. If you eat more, then the amount of calories and nutrients you get from that item will be higher. If you eat less, the amount will be lower.

Calories from fat. Use this information to compare products and to add up the amount of fat you eat. Limit fat to about 65 grams a day. This amount keeps fat at the recommended level—less than 30 percent of your daily calories, based on a 2,000-calorie (8,400-kilojoule) diet.

Nutrition Facts

Serving size ½ cup (114 g)
Servings per container 4

Amount per serving	
Calories 90	Calories from fat 30

	Percent Daily Value*
Total fat 3 g	5%
Saturated fat 0 g	0%
Cholesterol 0 mg	0%
Sodium 300 mg	13%
Total carbohydrate 13 g	4%
Dietary fiber 3 g	12%
Sugars 3 g	
Protein 3 g	

Vitamin A	80%	Vitamin C	60%
Calcium	4%	Iron	4%

*Percent Daily Values are based on a 2,000-calorie diet. Your daily values may be higher or lower depending on your calorie needs:

	Calories	2,000	2,500
Total fat	Less than	65 g	80 g
Saturated fat	Less than	20 g	25 g
Cholesterol	Less than	300 mg	300 mg
Sodium	Less than	2,400 mg	2,400 mg
Total carbohydrate		300 g	375 g
Fiber		25 g	30 g

Calories per gram:
Fat 9   Carbohydrates 4   Protein 4

Daily value. These values represent the amounts of nutrients and fiber desirable in 2,000- and 2,500-calorie (8,400- and 10,500-kilojoule) diets. The % Daily Value tells you how much of the recommended daily amount 1 serving contains, based on 2,000 calories (8,400 kilojoules).

For fat, saturated fat, cholesterol and sodium, choose foods with a low % Daily Value. For total carbohydrate, dietary fiber, vitamins and minerals, try to reach or exceed 100 percent of each.

Stocking your kitchen

You're more likely to prepare healthful dishes if you have everything you need at your fingertips. You don't need unusual or hard-to-find foods to eat well. You should be able to find everything you need at a well-stocked supermarket.

Here are examples of good foods to stock up on when you're grocery shopping:

Dairy products
Low-fat or fat-free milk
Low-fat or reduced-fat cottage cheese or ricotta
Reduced-fat cheeses
Reduced-fat or fat-free sour cream
Tub or squeeze margarine

Grains
Bread, bagels, pita bread
Low-fat flour tortillas
Plain cereal, dry or cooked
Rice, brown or white
Pasta, noodles and spaghetti

Fruit
Standard fresh varieties
Seasonal fresh fruits
Canned fruit in juice or water
Frozen fruit without added sugar
Dried fruit

Vegetables
Standard fresh varieties
Seasonal fresh vegetables
Frozen vegetables without added butter or sauces
Canned tomato products low in sodium
Canned vegetables or vegetable soups low in sodium

Legumes (without added salt)
Lentils
Black beans
Red (kidney) beans
Navy beans
Chickpeas (garbanzo beans)

Meat
White meat, skinless chicken and turkey
Fish (unbreaded)
Pork tenderloin
Extra-lean ground beef
Round or sirloin beef cuts

Baking items
Imitation butter, flakes or buds
Nonstick cooking spray
Canned evaporated milk, fat-free or reduced-fat
Cocoa powder, unsweetened
Angel food cake mix

Condiments, seasonings and spreads
Low-fat or fat-free salad dressings
Herbs
Spices
Flavored vinegars
Salsa or picante sauce

Healthful cooking techniques

Like a delicious meal, nutrition is the result of good ingredients that you carefully select and prepare. There's nothing unusual or complicated about cooking techniques for eating well. The difficult part is often just breaking away from habits that have become ingrained in your cooking routine.

To manage high blood pressure and improve your health, try to cook with less salt and little or no oils or other fats.

Here are some tips to get you started:

- To enhance a food's flavor without adding salt or fat, use onions, herbs, spices, colorful fresh peppers, fresh garlic, fresh ginger, fresh lemons and limes, flavored vinegars, sherry or other wines and reduced-sodium soy sauce.
- Dress up vegetables with flavored herbs, spices or butter-flavored powders, instead of salt or butter.
- Cut the amount of meat in stews and casseroles by a third and add more vegetables, rice or pasta.
- In recipes, substitute lower-fat dairy products, such as reduced-fat cream cheese and sour cream, for their higher-fat counterparts.
- To replace all or part of the sugar in recipes, use cinnamon, nutmeg, vanilla and fruit. They enhance sweetness.
- Invest in nonstick cookware to sauté or brown foods without adding fat. If you normally add a tablespoon of vegetable oil to a skillet, you can save 120 calories (504 kilojoules) and 14 grams of fat by using a nonstick skillet instead. Or use a vegetable oil cooking spray. It only adds about 1 gram of fat and few calories.
- Sauté onions, mushrooms or celery in a small amount of wine, low-sodium broth or water instead of butter or oil.
- Grill, broil, poach, roast or stir-fry your foods instead of always frying them.
- Cook fish in parchment paper or foil. This seals in flavor and juices.

Check out Mayo Clinic Health Oasis for healthful recipes
Visit our Web site at *www.mayohealth.org* to browse through great-tasting recipes that are low in fat and sodium and rich in nutrients. You can find the recipes in the Nutrition Center.

Eating well when eating out

Eating more healthfully doesn't confine you to eating at home. You can eat nutritiously away from home too. In fact, dining out can be a great opportunity to enjoy a variety of nutritious meals, without having to prepare them yourself.

Many restaurants provide healthful food choices. Some restaurants even reserve a special section of their menu for more healthful fare. For those restaurants that don't, keep in mind that many restaurants will honor special requests to prepare an item with less fat and sodium.

If the entrée is larger than you want, ask if you can have the lunch portion, even if you're eating dinner. You can also request a doggie bag when the meal is served. This way you can reserve half of the meal for the next day. Or, you might choose an appetizer for an entrée or split a meal with a companion.

What to order

Following these suggestions will help you keep your eating plan on target when you're away from home:

Appetizer. Choose appetizers with vegetables, fruit or fish, such as chopped, raw vegetables, fresh-fruit compote or shrimp cocktail (use lemon juice instead of cocktail sauce).

Soup. Broth or tomato-based soups are often high in sodium. Creamed soups, chowders, pureed soups and some fruit soups contain heavy cream and egg yolks. You're often better off avoiding soup and choosing fruit or a salad.

Salad. Order lettuce or spinach salads with dressings on the side. Caesar and Greek salads are high in fat, cholesterol and sodium. Chef salads are also high in fat, cholesterol and calories because of the amount of cheese, eggs and meat they contain. Taco salads typically aren't a good choice because they contain high-fat items such as cheese, guacamole, ground beef and a fried shell.

Bread. If you're offered a bread basket, choose bread, rolls, bread sticks or bagels. Eat them plain or with a little honey, jam or jelly. These fat-free toppings contribute few calories when used sparingly. Muffins, garlic toast or croissants have more fat. Crackers can be high in sodium.

Side dish. Choose a baked potato, boiled new potatoes, steamed vegetables, rice or fresh fruit instead of french fries, potato chips, onion rings or mayonnaise-based salads, such as potato salad. Ask that no butter or margarine be used to prepare the vegetable or rice.

Entrée. Look for entrées with descriptions that indicate low-fat content, such as London broil, grilled chicken breast, lemon-baked fish or broiled beef kabobs.

Avoid items with descriptions indicating higher-fat content, such as prime rib of beef, veal parmigiana, stuffed shrimp, fried chicken or filet mignon with béarnaise sauce.

When eating pasta, choose pasta with red or clam sauces. Skip pasta with meat or cheese stuffing or white sauces that contain bacon, butter, cream or eggs.

Dessert. Choose fresh fruit, poached spiced fruit, plain cake with fruit puree, sorbet or sherbet.

Alcohol. Alcohol is high in fat and calories. Excessive alcohol can also increase your blood pressure. If you choose to drink alcohol, limit the amount to one drink per day if you're a woman or smaller man and two drinks if you're a man. Alcohol's relationship to high blood pressure is discussed further in Chapter 8 (page 112).

Dining at ethnic restaurants

You don't have to limit yourself to standard American cuisine when eating out. You can eat a healthful meal at ethnic restaurants as well.

As with American foods, the problem to sidestep is excess fat and sodium. Sometimes fat or sodium is inherent in a country's culinary style. Other times, ethnic dishes simply gain fat or sodium in their American translation. Here's what you should know when eating these popular cuisines:

Chinese. The basis of Chinese food is low-fat ingredients such as vegetables and grains. To maintain these pluses, avoid fried dishes and extra-large portions. Choose items that are steamed or contain the words Jum (poached), Chu (boiled), Kow (roasted) or Shu (barbecued).

Avoid fried items such as crispy wonton appetizers or egg rolls. In addition, choose entrées containing chicken or seafood. Or, better yet, order a vegetarian dish.

Many Chinese foods are made with salty sauces, such as soy sauce, or with salty flavor enhancers, such as monosodium glutamate (MSG). Request the sauce on the side or ask that the item be made without soy sauce or MSG.

Italian. The foundation of many dishes is low-fat pasta. The key is not to cover it with rich sauces. Choose pasta with red or clam sauces.

Fresh tomato-based sauces also help you meet your daily vegetable requirements. Also look for simply prepared fish and chicken dishes. Good choices include chicken in wine sauce, grilled fish or shrimp marinara.

Avoid items that contain cream sauces, such as fettucine alfredo, or plenty of cheese, such as lasagna. Also avoid items with pancetta or prosciutto, Italian bacon and ham that are high in salt. If you like pizza, ask that it be prepared with less cheese and meat and more vegetables.

Mexican. Many Mexican restaurants—especially those north of the border—feature items high in fat. But you still can eat healthfully in a Mexican restaurant, if you choose well.

Select items that don't contain a lot of add-ons, such as cheese, sour cream or guacamole. Also choose items that aren't fried. Your best choices include fajitas, burritos or soft tacos. Fajitas are an especially good choice because you form them yourself. Instead of guacamole and sour cream, pile on more grilled vegetables and salsa. Salsa is fat-free and contains nutritious tomatoes and peppers.

Request black beans instead of refried beans. Black beans are lower in fat. If you can, request plain rice. Mexican rice can sometimes contain a high amount of sodium. Instead of snacking on fried chips and salsa before your meal, request plain tortillas to dip into your salsa.

Japanese. Japanese dishes contain mainly fish, rice and vegetables—foods high in nutrients. However, Japanese food also tends to be extremely salty. To limit sodium, stay away from items containing soy and other salty sauces. If you're not sure how the item is prepared, ask.

New American. These restaurants, which often feature Mediterranean, Pacific Rim or American Southwest cooking, generally offer a variety of healthful selections.

Seafood is a common dish. Ask for it broiled with lemon and herbs, which bring out its flavor. Items that are pan-roasted are also a good choice. The meat is browned quickly over very high heat, sealing in the juices and reducing the need for fat or sauces. Items rubbed with herbs also tend to be flavorful and contain less fat and salt.

Putting it all in perspective

If all the suggestions for eating well in this chapter seem a bit overwhelming, remember that eating well isn't an all-or-nothing approach.

Every food you eat doesn't need to be an excellent source of nutrients or fiber. It's also OK to eat high-fat or salty foods on occasion. But try to eat foods that promote your health more often than foods that don't. Over time, this approach to eating well will become a habit, and good habits can be as difficult to break as bad ones.

Wrap-up

Key points to remember from this chapter:
- A healthful diet can reduce your blood pressure as much as some medications.
- The DASH diet can help lower blood pressure by promoting generous amounts of whole grains, fruits, vegetables and low-fat dairy products. The diet is low in fat and rich in potassium, calcium and magnesium, nutrients associated with lower blood pressure.
- It's easier to eat well when you plan your meals, read food labels and stock up on healthful ingredients.
- When cooking, use less salt and little or no fats or oils. Look for other ways to enhance the flavor of your food.
- When eating out, look for dishes low in fat and sodium, and don't be afraid to make special requests.

Chapter 7

The Shakedown on Salt

Of all the issues related to high blood pressure, none is more controversial than salt—more specifically, the sodium in salt. Since the 1970s, health organizations have advised Americans—especially those with high blood pressure—to limit their intake of sodium. The recommendation stems from studies showing that a reduction in sodium can lower your blood pressure if you're "sodium-sensitive."

But what if you're not sodium-sensitive? And how should you interpret more recent studies suggesting that your weight and other aspects of your diet may be more important than limiting sodium?

In this chapter, we give you insights into the relationship between sodium and blood pressure. You'll learn how sodium can affect blood pressure and why controlling it can help you manage high blood pressure. And we'll tell you why avoiding excessive sodium is reasonable and safe for everyone.

Sodium's role

Sodium is an essential mineral. Its main role is to help maintain the right balance of fluids in your body. It also helps transmit nerve impulses that influence contraction and relaxation of your muscles.

You get sodium from the foods you eat. Many foods naturally contain some sodium. However, most sodium comes from sodium compounds

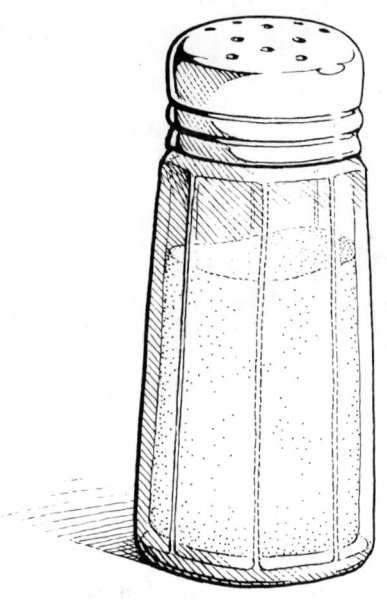

Sodium sources

1% drinking water
11% table/cooking salt
11% naturally inherent in food
77% processed foods

added to food during commercial processing and meal preparation at home (see Sodium-based food additives). Salt (sodium chloride) is the most common source of sodium. It's made up of 40 percent sodium and 60 percent chloride.

You need a minimum of 500 milligrams (mg) of sodium each day. That's a little more than 11/44 teaspoon of salt. However, most Americans consume 3,000 to 4,000 mg of sodium daily.

Your kidneys regulate the amount of sodium in your body. When your sodium levels are low, they conserve sodium. When your levels are high, they excrete the excess amount in your urine.

Sometimes, though, your kidneys can't eliminate enough sodium. Extra sodium starts to accumulate in your blood, and because sodium attracts and holds water, your blood volume increases. Your heart has to work harder to move the increased volume of blood through your blood vessels, increasing pressure on your arteries. Heart, kidney, liver and lung disease can all lead to an inability to regulate sodium. In addition, some people are simply more sensitive to the presence of high levels of sodium in their blood.

Sodium sensitivity

How people react to sodium varies. Some people—both healthy adults and people with high blood pressure—can consume as much sodium as they like and it has no or little effect on their blood pressure.

For others, too much sodium quickly leads to an increase in blood pressure, often triggering the development of high blood pressure. This condition is referred to as sodium or salt sensitivity.

Sodium-based food additives

These sodium compounds are commonly added to food during processing and cooking.

Salt (sodium chloride)
   Used in cooking or at the table; used in canning and preserving

Monosodium glutamate (MSG)
   A flavor enhancer used in home and restaurant cooking and in many packaged, canned and frozen foods

Baking soda (sodium bicarbonate)
   Sometimes used to leaven breads and cakes; sometimes added to vegetables in cooking; used as an alkalizer for indigestion

Baking powder
   A mixture of baking soda, starch and an acid used to leaven quick breads and cakes

Disodium phosphate
   Present in some quick-cooking cereals and processed cheeses

Sodium alginate
   Used in many chocolate milks and ice creams to make a smooth mixture

Sodium benzoate
   Used as a preservative in many condiments such as relishes, sauces and salad dressings

Sodium hydroxide
   Used in food processing to soften and loosen skins of ripe olives and certain fruits and vegetables

Sodium nitrate
   Used in cured meats and sausages

Sodium propionate
   Used in pasteurized cheese and in some breads and cakes to inhibit growth of molds

Sodium sulfite
   Used to bleach certain fruits such as maraschino cherries and glazed or crystallized fruits that are to be artificially colored; used as a preservative in some dried fruits such as prunes

From Sodium and Blood Pressure, American Heart Association, 1996. By permission.

Approximately 40 percent of people with high blood pressure are sodium-sensitive. The condition is more common in blacks of African-American descent and adults age 65 or older. In addition, people with diabetes tend to be more sensitive to high levels of sodium. Exactly what causes sodium sensitivity isn't known. Genetics may play a role in some cases, especially among blacks.

There's no easy way to tell if you're sodium-sensitive, other than to limit your consumption of sodium and see if doing so lowers your blood pressure. Medical tests can pinpoint your response to varying levels of sodium, but testing isn't practical or necessary.

If you're sensitive to sodium, following a low-sodium diet will likely produce a noticeable reduction in your blood pressure. If you have high blood pressure, your doctor also may recommend a diuretic medication that eliminates excess fluid from your blood. Even if you take a diuretic, you still need to avoid too much sodium. If you don't, the drug may cause you to lose excessive amounts of other essential minerals, such as potassium and magnesium.

Current recommendation

The National High Blood Pressure Education Program, sponsored by the National Institutes of Health, recommends that all Americans limit sodium to 2,400 mg a day. That's equivalent to about a teaspoon of salt.

Many health professionals and organizations, including doctors in Mayo Clinic's Division of Hypertension, support this recommendation. Here's why:
- If you have high blood pressure and you're sodium-sensitive, reducing sodium can lower your blood pressure. Limiting sodium in combination with other lifestyle changes, such as following a healthful diet and increasing your activity level, may be enough to keep you from having to take medication to control your blood pressure.
- If you're taking blood pressure medication, limiting sodium can help increase the effectiveness of the drug.
- If you're at risk for high blood pressure, limiting sodium along with other lifestyle changes may help prevent development of the disease.
- If you're healthy, limiting sodium as part of a healthful diet is safe

and reasonable. In addition, it may keep you from becoming at risk for the disease as you get older, when high blood pressure is more prevalent and your sensitivity to sodium often increases.

Although it hasn't been proven that reducing sodium will reduce your risk for high blood pressure, large population studies show that when people cut back on sodium their blood pressures decrease. There are also fewer deaths from heart attack and stroke. This suggests that the average person—especially one with a family history of high blood pressure—may benefit from reducing sodium.

The controversy

Since the recommendation that all Americans should limit sodium was made 30 years ago, it's been a source of controversy—mainly because much of the data related to sodium and high blood pressure aren't clear-cut and can be interpreted differently. In addition, results of more recent studies haven't helped end the debate.

Three main issues are feeding the controversy:
- Studies show that when some people with normal blood pressure cut back on sodium, their blood pressure decreases very little, if at all.
- Recent studies suggest losing weight and eating a diet that emphasizes grains, fruits, vegetables, low-fat dairy products and moderate levels of sodium may be more important for managing blood pressure than limiting sodium alone.
- A 1998 study published in the medical journal *The Lancet* found that people who ate very little sodium had more heart attacks years later than people who consumed more sodium. At least one other earlier study also reached a similar conclusion.

Officials with the National High Blood Pressure Education Program continue to monitor all of the scientific information regarding sodium and blood pressure. Their position is that the bulk of evidence suggests that avoiding sodium is reasonable and safe. They also believe that for people who are sodium-sensitive, sodium control is as important as other lifestyle factors, including a nutritious diet and losing weight. In addition, although restricting sodium may benefit some people only minimally, for the nation as a whole, it can have a major impact in terms of preventing future disease and reducing stroke and heart attacks related to high blood pressure.

What you should do

If your doctor or a registered dietitian has suggested that you cut back on sodium to lower your blood pressure, it's advice you should follow. Even if you haven't been told to reduce sodium, you should try to limit the amount you eat each day.

There are several ways you can reduce sodium in your diet:

Eat more fresh and fewer processed foods. Fresh foods usually have less sodium than processed ones. Most fresh vegetables are naturally low in sodium. Canned vegetables and vegetable juices, such as tomato juice, usually have added salt. Fruits are generally low in sodium, whether they're fresh, frozen or canned.

Fresh meat is lower in sodium than luncheon meat, bacon, hot dogs, sausage and ham. All these foods have sodium added to flavor and help preserve them.

Soups, frozen dinners and other fast-food items typically have salt added when they're prepared. Snacks, such as potato chips, corn chips, pretzels, popcorn, crackers and nuts, often have a large amount of added salt. It's best to eat them sparingly.

Look for lower-sodium products. Some processed foods that are high in sodium are also prepared in lower-sodium versions. These include soups, broths, canned vegetables and vegetable juices, processed lean meats, ketchup and soy sauce.

Just because a food is low in fat or calories doesn't mean it's low in sodium. Sometimes extra sodium is added to low-fat products to increase their flavor.

Read labels. The Nutrition Facts label tells you how much sodium is in each serving. It also lists whether salt or sodium–containing compounds are ingredients. If sodium is one of the first three

> **Retraining your taste buds**
>
> A low-sodium diet may taste bland for a few weeks, but your taste buds will eventually adapt to your change in diet. A taste for salt isn't something you're born with, it's something you acquire. Just as you taught your taste buds to enjoy salt, you can teach them to appreciate less salty foods.
>
> As you use less salt, your preference for salt will lessen, allowing you to enjoy the taste of the food itself. Most people find that after a few weeks of limiting sodium they no longer miss salt.

Spice it up

It's easy to make food taste good without using salt. Here are suggestions for herbs, spices and flavorings you can use to enhance the flavor of certain foods.

Meat, poultry, fish

Beef	Bay leaf, dry mustard, marjoram, nutmeg, onion, pepper, sage, thyme
Chicken	Dill, ginger, oregano, paprika, parsley, rosemary, sage, tarragon, thyme
Fish	Bay leaf, curry powder, dry mustard, lemon juice, paprika
Lamb	Cranberry, curry powder, garlic, rosemary
Pork	Cranberry, garlic, onion, oregano, pepper, sage
Veal	Bay leaf, curry powder, ginger, oregano

Vegetables

Broccoli	Lemon juice, oregano
Carrots	Cinnamon, cloves, nutmeg, rosemary, sage
Cauliflower	Nutmeg, tarragon
Corn	Chives, cumin, green pepper, paprika, parsley, fresh tomatoes
Green beans	Dill, unsalted French dressing, lemon juice, nutmeg, tarragon
Peas	Mint, onion, parsley
Potatoes	Dill, garlic, chopped green pepper, onion, parsley, sage
Tomatoes	Basil, dill, onion, oregano, parsley, sage

Low-sodium soups

Creamed	Bay leaf, dill, paprika, peppercorns, tarragon
Vegetable	Basil, bay leaf, curry, dill, garlic, onion, oregano

Other

Cottage cheese	Caraway seeds, cayenne, chives, dill
Popcorn	Curry, garlic powder, onion powder
Rice	Basil, cumin, curry, green pepper, oregano
Salads	Basil, dill, lemon juice, parsley, vinegar

ingredients listed, the product is high in sodium. Also look for other sources of sodium, such as monosodium glutamate (MSG), baking soda or baking powder.

Some over-the-counter medications also contain large amounts of sodium. They include some antacids, alkalizers (Alka-Seltzer, Bromo Seltzer), laxatives and cough medicines. If you use such a product frequently, check the label or ask your pharmacist to find out its sodium content. Try to purchase brands of these products that are sodium-free. If that isn't possible, talk with your doctor about other possible medications that contain less sodium.

Don't add salt to food when cooking. Instead, use spices, herbs, pepper, fresh lemon, onion, fresh garlic, sherry and other wines to add flavor to your food. Check the label on the spices to make sure they don't contain sodium.

Don't add salt at the table. If you think your food needs more flavor, try another seasoning, such as lemon, pepper or a sodium-free herb blend.

Limit your use of condiments. Salad dressings, sauces, dips,

Making sense of sodium claims

You'll find sodium-related claims on many foods. Here's what they mean:

Sodium-free. Each serving contains less than 5 milligrams (mg) of sodium.

Very low-sodium. Each serving contains 35 mg of sodium or less.

Low-sodium. Each serving contains 140 mg of sodium or less.

Lite or light in sodium. The sodium content has been reduced by at least 50 percent.

Reduced-sodium. The product contains at least 25 percent less sodium than the original.

Unsalted or without added salt. No salt is added during processing of a food that normally contains salt. However, some foods with these claims may still be high in sodium.

As a general rule, Mayo Clinic registered dietitians suggest that you plan most of your meals around foods that contain no more than 200 mg of sodium in a serving. For main-dish items, look for those that don't exceed 600 mg of sodium per meal.

ketchup, mustard and relish all contain sodium. As you use less salt, you may be tempted to use more condiments. Pickles and olives contain a very high amount of sodium.

Rinse canned foods. Rinsing canned vegetables and meats helps remove some of the sodium. But don't rely on this as a way to reduce sodium. Rinsing only removes about one-third of the sodium. It's better to purchase fresh or low-sodium versions.

Your sodium guide

The DASH diet discussed in the previous chapter outlines the foods and number of servings you should eat to reduce your blood pressure. The following guide is meant to complement the DASH diet. It lists foods that are low in sodium and can be eaten more frequently and high-sodium foods that you should avoid or eat only occasionally.

If you're trying to lose weight, a registered dietitian can adapt the guidelines to meet your specific calorie requirement.

Meat and meat substitutes

Use:
- Fresh and frozen beef, pork, lamb, veal, poultry and wild game
- Fresh or frozen fish, shrimp, scallops and clams (unbreaded and not packed in brine or salt)
- Cheese labeled low-sodium or salt-free
- Cottage cheese, dry curd or low-sodium
- Eggs
- No-salt-added peanut butter or unsalted nuts
- No-salt-added canned tuna or other seafood
- Frozen and microwave dinners that have less than 600 milligrams (mg) sodium per dinner

Limit (2 or 3 times per week):
- Regular cottage cheese and mild aged natural cheese (such as brick, Monterey Jack, mild cheddar)
- Regular peanut butter or peanuts containing salt
- Canned tuna and other canned seafood packed with 50 percent to 60 percent less salt than usual
- Reduced-sodium processed meats and cheeses
- Lobster and crab

Avoid:
- Meat, fish or poultry that is salt-cured, canned with salt or smoked (such as bacon, chipped beef, corned beef, wieners, ham, luncheon meats and sausages)
- Processed cheese and cheese spreads
- Pickled herring, eggs and meats
- Salted nuts
- Frozen and microwave dinners that have more than 600 mg sodium per dinner

Fats and oils
Use:
- Oil, margarine or butter
- Low-sodium salad dressing
- Shortening, mayonnaise and unsalted gravy
- Cream cheese, sour cream

Avoid:
- Salad dressings, gravies, spreads and sauces with more than 180 mg of sodium per serving

Milk
Use:
- Milk (fat-free, low-fat, reduced-fat or whole) and yogurt

Limit (2 or 3 times per week):
- Commercially cultured buttermilk
- Instant mixes with more than 200 mg sodium per serving

Grains and starches
Use:
- Grains with less than 180 mg sodium per serving (such as bread, dinner rolls, bagels, English muffins, cereals)
- Quick breads such as pancakes or biscuits made from home recipes
- Plain muffins
- Crackers with unsalted tops, graham crackers or melba toast
- Potatoes, rice or pasta
- Unsalted popcorn, pretzels or chips
- Low-sodium canned soups, bouillon and broth

Avoid:
- Grains with more than 180 mg sodium per serving
- Quick breads such as pancakes and biscuits made from commercial mixes
- Salted popcorn
- Regular canned soups, dried soup mixes, broth and bouillon
- Commercially canned and frozen convenience foods (unless labeled low-sodium)
- Commercially prepared refrigerator dough

Vegetables

Use:
- Fresh, unsalted frozen vegetables or no-salt-added canned vegetables
- No-salt-added tomato juice and vegetable juice cocktail, no-salt-added canned tomato products

Avoid:
- Canned salted tomato products
- Commercially canned and frozen vegetables with added salt, sauce or breading
- Salted tomato juice and vegetable juice cocktail
- Sauerkraut and pickled vegetables

Fruits

Use:
- Fresh, frozen and canned fruit

Avoid:
- Fruits dried with a sodium compound

Desserts and sweets

Use:
- Homemade desserts, cooked pudding and box mixes with less than 200 mg sodium per serving
- Fresh fruit, gelatin, fruit ice, sherbet, plain cake, meringue, ice cream and frozen yogurt
- Jams, jelly, honey
- Hard candy, jelly beans

Avoid:
- Box mixes (such as cakes, muffins, cookies) with more than 200 mg sodium per serving
- Desserts and candies prepared with salted nuts
- Refrigerator dough and commercial coffee cakes
- Instant pudding and pie filling mixes, cream or fruit pies

Beverages
Use:
- Water
- Fruit juices or fruit drinks, lemonade
- Decaffeinated and regular coffee and tea

Limit (1 to 2 servings per day):
- Cocoa (made with cocoa powder)
- Sweetened or sugar-free carbonated beverages

Tap water:
- Sodium content varies with the local water supply. Chemically softened water may contain added sodium. Discuss use of softened water with a registered dietitian

Avoid:
- Cocktail beverage mixes, instant beverage mixes such as instant cocoa, commercial sport drinks

Note: Choose beverages with less than 70 mg sodium per serving

Seasonings and condiments
Use:
- Herbs, spices and salt-free herb/spice mixes
- Garlic powder, onion powder and pepper
- Salt-free bouillon cubes or granules
- Unsalted ketchup, mustard and barbecue sauce
- Lemon juice, flavoring extracts and vinegar
- Prepared horseradish
- Table wine (not cooking wine)

Limit (1 or 2 times per week):
- Regular ketchup or mustard, 1 tbsp.
- Regular bottled meat and barbecue sauces, 1 tbsp.
- Commercial salsa, 1-2 tbsp.

Avoid:
- "Light salt" products, seasoning salts and mixes (such as celery salt, garlic salt, onion salt)
- Meat tenderizer
- Olives and pickles
- Soy sauce, teriyaki sauce and monosodium glutamate (MSG)
- Cooking wine

About salt substitutes

Before you try a salt substitute, check with your doctor.

Some salt substitutes or "lite" salts contain a mixture of sodium chloride (salt) and other compounds. To achieve that familiar salty taste, you may end up using more of the salt substitute than you do regular salt, and the result is that you don't reduce your sodium intake at all.

In addition, potassium chloride is a common ingredient in salt substitutes. Too much potassium can be harmful if you have kidney problems or you're taking certain medications to treat high blood pressure or heart failure. Potassium-sparing diuretic drugs cause your kidneys to retain potassium. If you take a potassium-sparing diuretic and use a salt substitute containing potassium, too much potassium can build up in your body. Possible side effects include potentially life-threatening heart rhythm disturbances.

Wrap-up

Key points to remember from this chapter:
- Sodium significantly increases blood pressure in people who are sensitive to it.
- Approximately 40 percent of people with high blood pressure are sodium-sensitive. You're more likely to be sodium-sensitive if you're black, age 65 or older or have diabetes.
- Whether you have high blood pressure or are healthy, limiting sodium to 2,400 milligrams daily is reasonable and safe.
- Processed foods generally contain the most sodium. Fresh foods tend to be lower in sodium.
- Instead of salt, use herbs, spices and other flavorings to enhance the flavor of foods.
- Don't use a salt substitute without first talking with your doctor. A salt substitute isn't recommended if you have kidney disease or if you're taking certain medications for high blood pressure or heart failure.

Chapter 8

Tobacco, Alcohol and Caffeine

Every day, millions of people sit back and relax for a few minutes with a cigarette. And odds are that you're part of the great majority who occasionally has an alcoholic drink or regularly indulges in a cup of caffeinated coffee or tea or a caffeinated soft drink.

Even if you're healthy, tobacco, alcohol and caffeine can raise your blood pressure to an unhealthful level. But if you have high blood pressure, or you're at risk for it, you need to be especially alert to the effect that these substances can have on your blood pressure.

Clearly, smoking is dangerous. If you want to reduce your risk for complications from high blood pressure, don't smoke. Alcohol and caffeine, however, are pleasures that most people with high blood pressure can continue to enjoy—but in moderation.

Tobacco and high blood pressure

Approximately one out of three people with high blood pressure smokes. Simply having high blood pressure puts you at increased risk for a heart attack or stroke. But if you have high blood pressure and you smoke, you're three to five times more likely to die of a heart attack or heart failure than someone who doesn't smoke. In addition, you're more than twice as likely to die of a stroke.

How smoking affects blood pressure

The nicotine in tobacco is what causes your blood pressure to increase shortly after you take that first puff. Nicotine, like many other chemicals in tobacco smoke, is picked up by tiny blood vessels in your lungs and distributed into your bloodstream. It takes only about 10 seconds for nicotine to reach your brain. Your brain reacts to nicotine by signaling your adrenal glands to release epinephrine (adrenaline). This powerful hormone narrows your blood vessels, forcing your heart to pump harder under higher pressure.

After smoking just two cigarettes, both systolic and diastolic pressures increase an average of about 10 mm Hg. Your blood pressure remains at this increased level for about 30 minutes after you finish smoking. As the effects of the nicotine wear off, your blood pressure gradually decreases. However, if you smoke heavily, your blood pressure is at a high level throughout most of the day.

In addition to promoting the release of adrenaline, smoking has other damaging effects. The chemicals in tobacco can scar the inner walls of your arteries, leaving them more susceptible to accumulation of cholesterol-containing fatty deposits (plaque) that narrow your arteries. Tobacco also triggers the release of hormones that cause your body to retain fluid. Both of these factors—narrowed arteries and increased fluid—can lead to high blood pressure.

Why quitting is crucial

Stopping smoking may reduce your blood pressure by only a few points. But doing so is important for two reasons.

First, quitting smoking may increase the effectiveness of your medication. Smoking interferes with some blood pressure medications, keeping them from working as well as they can, or working at all.

Second, and more importantly, stopping smoking greatly reduces your risk for a heart attack, heart failure or stroke. Having high blood pressure puts you at increased risk for these conditions because of the damage it can cause to your arteries. Blood supply to your heart and brain may be reduced. Plus, your risk for formation of a blood clot increases.

Smoking also damages your arteries and produces the same cardiovascular risks. Therefore, when you combine high blood pressure with smoking, your odds for a heart attack, heart failure or stroke are much greater.

> **Quitters do win**
>
> Many people continue to smoke because they figure they can't undo the damage already done to their bodies. Or they figure that quitting is hopeless—they know too many smokers who tried to stop and failed. Some people also believe that stopping smoking will doom them to weight gain. All these assumptions are wrong.
>
> As for your body, it has an incredible ability to repair itself. By the end of your first nonsmoking year, your risk of heart attack begins to decrease, and after 5 years it's almost the same as that for people who've never smoked. In addition, after 10 to 15 years your risk of getting lung cancer and other cancers associated with tobacco use is about the same as that in people who never smoked.
>
> It's true that about 75 percent of smokers aren't able to stop on their first attempt. But stopping smoking is like learning anything else new. It often takes several attempts, and one bad experience shouldn't keep you from trying again. In fact, you can learn from previous attempts, increasing your chances for being successful in the future.
>
> It's also true that some people gain weight after they stop smoking. However, the amount is usually small. On average, most people gain around 5 pounds (2.3 kilograms).

Breaking tobacco's grip

There's no one perfect plan for quitting smoking. Some people can simply stop and never smoke again. For others, quitting takes several tries and various approaches.

But you can quit—many people have. Following these steps can increase your chances for being successful.

Step 1: Do your homework. That way you'll know what to expect. You may experience physical withdrawal symptoms for at least 10 days. Common symptoms include irritability, anxiety and loss of concentration. Afterward, you may still have an urge to light up in familiar smoking situations, such as after a meal or while driving. These urges are generally very brief, but they can be very strong.

By knowing what to expect and having alternative activities planned, you'll be better prepared to handle the urges. These activities might include chewing gum after a meal or snacking on some carrot sticks or low-salt pretzels while driving to keep your hands busy.

Most relapses take place within 4 weeks after quitting smoking. Often, the relapse occurs not only because of the power of nicotine addiction but also because the smoker didn't have a well-conceived quitting plan.

Step 2: Set a stop date. Quitting cold turkey seems to work better than cutting down gradually. So carefully select a date to quit smoking. Don't try to quit when you know your stress level will be high.

Many smokers choose to quit during a relaxing vacation. One reason is that your routine changes on vacation, so it's easier to break free of smoking rituals than when you're at work or home.

Step 3: Tell others about your decision. Having the support of family, friends and coworkers can help you reach your goal more quickly. However, many smokers keep their plans to quit a secret. That's because they don't want to look like a failure if they go back to smoking.

Remember, it takes many people three or more tries before they're successful. So there's no reason to feel like a failure just because your effort may not work out this time. Enlisting the help of at least one person can enhance your chances of success.

Step 4: Start changing your routine. Before your stop date, cut down on the number of places you smoke. For instance, stop smoking in your car, and smoke in only one room of the house or outside. This approach will help reduce your smoking urges so you can be more comfortable in those places without smoking.

Step 5: Talk with your doctor about medications. Nicotine is a highly addictive substance. Withdrawal from nicotine can produce irritability, anxiety and difficulty concentrating. Medications are available that can help lessen withdrawal symptoms and increase your chances of being successful (see "Medications to help you quit").

Step 6: Take one day at a time. On your stop day, quit completely. Each day, focus your attention on remaining tobacco-free.

Medications to help you quit

The medications listed below can reduce the difficult side effects of nicotine withdrawal and make quitting smoking easier. Use them according to your doctor's instructions, gradually tapering their use over a period of weeks to months.

Nicotine patches. Available as over-the-counter products and by prescription, the nicotine patch is placed on your skin, where it gradually releases nicotine into your body. This helps reduce nicotine cravings when you cut back or stop smoking. The patches can irritate your skin, but you can minimize the irritation by rotating the site of the patch and applying an over-the-counter cortisone cream.

Nicotine gum. You also can purchase over-the-counter nicotine gum. Bite into it a few times, then "park" it between your cheek and gum. The lining of your mouth absorbs the nicotine the gum releases. Nicotine gum can satisfy your nicotine urge, the same as the patch.

Nicotine nasal spray. It helps you quit in the same way as the patch or gum, but instead you spray nicotine into your nose. There, it's quickly absorbed into your bloodstream through the lining of your nose, providing a quicker response to nicotine cravings than the other products. It's intended mainly for when you need a quick "hit" of nicotine. The product is available only by prescription.

Nicotine inhaler. This relatively new medication is available only by prescription. The device looks like a plastic cigarette. One end of the inhaler has a plastic tip like that used on cigars. When you put this tip in your mouth and inhale, like puffing on a cigarette, the inhaler releases a nicotine vapor into your mouth, reducing your craving for nicotine. It also helps smokers who miss smoking's hand-to-mouth ritual.

Non-nicotine medication. Bupropion (Wellbutrin, Zyban) is the first non-nicotine medication approved by the Food and Drug Administration as a stop-smoking aid. It's not clear exactly how the drug works, but it stimulates the same chemicals involved in nicotine addiction. Bupropion is also available only by prescription.

Step 7: Avoid smoking situations. Change the situations in which you used to smoke. Leave the table immediately after meals if this is a time you used to light up. Take a walk instead. If you smoked while using the telephone, avoid long phone conversations or change the place where you talk. If you had a favorite smoking chair, avoid it.

You'll soon be able to anticipate when the urge to smoke will hit you. Before it hits, start doing something that makes smoking inconvenient, such as washing your car or mowing the lawn. Your smoking behavior is deeply ingrained and automatic. So you need to anticipate your reflex behavior and plan alternatives.

Step 8: Time each urge. Check your watch when a smoking urge hits. Most are short. Once you realize this, it's easier to resist. Remind yourself, "I can make it another few minutes and then the urge will pass."

Alcohol and high blood pressure

The best advice about alcohol is this—if you drink, do it in moderation.

Even for people with high blood pressure, small amounts of alcohol don't seem to increase blood pressure. And some evidence suggests that moderate drinking may reduce your risk of heart attack and boost your production of "good" (high-density lipoprotein, or HDL) cholesterol. HDL cholesterol helps protect your arteries from becoming narrowed or blocked by accumulation of plaque.

Excessive alcohol is the problem. It can increase your blood pressure and interfere with your medication. Heavy drinking is responsible for about 8 percent of all cases of high blood pressure in the United States.

What's "moderate" drinking?
It may be less than you think.

Alcoholic drinks contain various amounts of ethanol—the more ethanol, the stronger the drink. For most men, moderate drinking is no more than two drinks—1 ounce (30 milliliters) of ethanol—a day. Two drinks equates to two 12-ounce (360-mL) cans of beer, two 5-ounce (150-mL) glasses of wine or two 1-ounce (30-mL) shot glasses of 100-proof whiskey.

For women and small-framed men, moderate drinking is half that—one drink or no more than half an ounce (15 mL) of ethanol daily. The

> **Too much, too soon = too high**
> If you drink too much alcohol and you want to cut back, it's best to gradually reduce how much you drink over a period of 1 to 2 weeks.
>
> People who drink heavily and suddenly stop consuming alcohol can develop severe high blood pressure that lasts for several days. That's because when you suddenly remove alcohol from your blood, your body releases large amounts of epinephrine (adrenaline), which causes your blood pressure to rise sharply.
>
> If you have high blood pressure and you drink more than a moderate amount of alcohol, talk with your doctor about the safest and most successful way to limit or avoid alcohol.

amount is less because women and smaller-sized men generally absorb more ethanol.

How alcohol affects blood pressure

Exactly how excessive alcohol—more than a moderate amount—increases blood pressure is unknown. One theory is that it triggers the release of the hormone epinephrine (adrenaline), which narrows your blood vessels.

However, it's clear that reducing your consumption of alcohol can reduce your blood pressure. Excessive drinkers who cut back to moderate levels of alcohol consumption can lower their systolic blood pressure by about 5 mm Hg and their diastolic pressure about 3 mm Hg.

Combining a nutritious diet with reduced alcohol use can produce an even larger reduction—a drop of about 10 mm Hg in systolic pressure and 7 mm Hg in diastolic pressure. One reason for this effect is that people who consume too much alcohol generally don't get adequate amounts of nutrients that help control blood pressure, such as potassium, calcium and magnesium.

People on blood pressure medication who limit alcohol also tend to be more diligent about taking their medication. When influenced by alcohol, you may forget to take your pills or take them improperly.

Alcohol and blood pressure medications

Although it's OK to drink alcohol in moderation, if you take medication you may need to pay careful attention to when or how you consume alcohol. Alcohol can interfere with the effectiveness of some blood pressure medications and increase their side effects.

If you mix alcohol with a beta blocker, which relaxes your blood vessels and slows your heart rate, you may feel light-headed or faint—especially if you're a bit overheated or if you stand suddenly. You can experience the same symptoms if you drink alcohol near the time you take an angiotensin-converting enzyme (ACE) inhibitor, which widens your blood vessels, or certain calcium antagonists, which can slow your heart rate. If you do feel dizzy or faint, sit until the feeling passes. Drinking water will also help.

If you take a central-acting agent that works through your central nervous system, you could become unusually depressed after drinking alcohol. Both the medications and alcohol are sedatives.

Listen to your body. If you feel light-headed or depressed after a drink or two, talk with your doctor about how much alcohol you can safely drink and when.

Caffeine and high blood pressure

Found in coffee, tea, soft drinks and chocolate, caffeine is a mild stimulant that can fight fatigue, boost your concentration and lighten your mood. But if you use too much—something that's easy to do—caffeine can leave you jittery, cause your hands to tremble and possibly increase your blood pressure.

How caffeine affects blood pressure

Caffeine's influence on blood pressure is a topic of debate. Some studies have found that people who consume caffeine regularly throughout the day have a higher average blood pressure than if they didn't consume any. However, most studies have concluded that regular consumers of caffeine develop a tolerance to the stimulant. And afterwhile, it doesn't have any effect on their blood pressure.

It's clear, though, that among people who don't consume caffeine regularly or who consume more than they're used to, caffeine can cause a temporary but sharp rise in blood pressure.

Specifically what causes this spike in blood pressure is uncertain. Some researchers suggest that caffeine narrows your blood vessels by blocking the effects of adenosine (uh-DEN-o-seen), a natural hormone

Calculating your caffeine intake

If you have high blood pressure, limit caffeine to about 200 milligrams (mg) daily. Here are some common sources of caffeine and the amount of caffeine they contain:

Source	Caffeine (mg)
Coffee, ¾ cup (6 fl. oz./180 mL)	
Brewed, drip	103
Instant	57
Decaffeinated, brewed and instant	2
Espresso (single)	
Regular	100
Decaffeinated	5
Tea, ¾ cup (6 fl. oz./180 mL)	
Black, brewed 3 minutes	40
Instant	30
Decaffeinated	1
Soft drinks, 1½ cups (12 fl. oz./360 mL)	
Cola type, regular and diet	31-70
Non-cola type	0-55
Chocolate	
Cocoa, dry powder, 1 tbsp.	10
Baking chocolate, 1 oz. (30 g)	25
Chocolate milk, 1 cup (8 fl. oz./250 mL)	10
Milk chocolate bar, 1½ oz. (45 g)	10

From Bowes and Church's Food Values of Portions Commonly Used, 17th ed. Lippincott-Raven Publishers, 1998. By permission.

that helps keep them widened.

    As a precaution, many doctors caution people with high blood pressure to limit daily caffeine to no more than two cups of coffee, three or four cups of tea or two to four cans of caffeinated soda. Also avoid caffeine right before activities that naturally increase your blood pressure, such as exercise or hard physical labor.

Limiting caffeine is also good for your general health. Depending on your sensitivity to caffeine, even a couple of cups of coffee can affect your:

Nervous system. Too much caffeine can make you nervous, anxious or irritable. It also can worsen panic attacks and cause insomnia.

Digestive system. Caffeine can produce heartburn, constipation, diarrhea, gastrointestinal upset or irritate existing stomach ulcers.

Bladder. Caffeine can cause bladder irritation in some people. It's also a mild diuretic, causing you to urinate more.

> **Cut back slowly**
> If you plan to reduce caffeine, the best way is to taper the amount you drink over several weeks. This will help you avoid headaches and other side effects that can result when you drastically reduce your normal use of caffeine.

Wrap-up

Key points to remember from this chapter:
- If you have high blood pressure and you smoke, your risk of death from a heart attack or heart failure is at least three times higher, and your risk of death from stroke is at least two times higher, than if you didn't smoke.
- Medications designed to taper nicotine withdrawal can help you quit smoking.
- Eight percent of all cases of high blood pressure are due to excessive use of alcohol.
- Moderate alcohol use doesn't appear to affect blood pressure.
- Alcohol may increase the side effects of some high blood pressure medications.
- Caffeine can cause a temporary but sharp rise in blood pressure in some people.
- If you have high blood pressure, limit caffeine to two cups of coffee, three or four cups of tea or two to four cans of caffeinated soda daily.

Chapter 9

Managing Stress

If you lead a stressful life or you're a "type A" personality—competitive, intense, impatient—you're destined to have high blood pressure. This is a common belief. But it's not true. There are many type A individuals with normal blood pressure, just as there are relaxed people with high blood pressure.

Stress can increase your blood pressure temporarily. When you're scared, nervous or under a tight deadline, your blood pressure naturally increases. But in most cases, once you begin to relax, your blood pressure goes back down again.

If you have high blood pressure, simply reducing your stress level may not lower your blood pressure. But managing stress is important for other reasons. Less stress often results in the following:

Better control of blood pressure. The temporary increases in blood pressure caused by stress can make your high blood pressure more difficult to manage. When you're under less stress, lifestyle changes and medications may work more effectively.

A more positive attitude. Stress can interfere with and dampen your enthusiasm to take control of your blood pressure. It's easier to be physically active, eat healthfully, lose weight and limit alcohol when you're relaxed and happy.

There are many ways to manage stress. You may want to experiment with some different techniques until you find those stress relievers that fit your lifestyle and daily routine.

What is stress?

Think of stress as a spice. Too little spice results in a bland-tasting meal. Too much spice makes you sick. But when you use the correct amount, spice enhances flavor. Stress works in much the same way.

Stress can be negative or positive:

- Negative stress occurs when you feel out of control or under constant pressure. You may have trouble concentrating on a project. You may feel isolated from others. Family, finances, work and isolation are common causes of negative stress.
- Positive stress provides you with a feeling of excitement and opportunity. You feel confident when approaching a situation. Among athletes, positive stress often helps them perform better in competition than in practice. Other examples of positive stressors may include a new job or birth of a child.

Stress is also highly individualized. Some people cope well with difficult or tense situations. Others melt under the pressure. In addition, what's a "stressor" for one person may not cause stress in another.

The stress response

When dealing with a frightful event or an ongoing tension in your life, your body's physical response to any stressor is similar to a physical threat. Your body gears up to face the challenge ("fight") or muster enough strength to move out of trouble's way ("flight").

This "fight-or-flight" response results from the release of an assortment of hormones that cause your body to shift into overdrive. Among them are the hormones epinephrine (adrenaline) and cortisol, which cause your heart to beat faster and your blood pressure to increase.

Other physical changes also occur. More blood and nutrients are sent to your brain and muscles, and less to your skin. That's why you may look pale during moments of fright or high stress. Your body also releases fibrin, a chemical that makes your blood clot more easily. In a physical attack, this would help slow or stop a bleeding wound.

Your nervous system also springs into action. Your pupils dilate to enhance your vision. Your facial muscles tense up to make you look more intimidating. And you perspire more to cool your body.

Your body has many ways of letting you know when it's under too much stress. You may become discouraged, irritable, cynical, emotional or even reclusive. All of these emotions affect how you think, feel and act. However, these changes can sometimes be easy to miss because they may sneak up gradually, over a long time.

The physical symptoms aren't as easy to ignore. They may include a headache, stomach upset, insomnia, fatigue and frequent illness. You may find yourself reverting to nervous habits, such as biting your nails or smoking. You might even turn to alcohol or drugs.

Stress and blood pressure

The hormones epinephrine (adrenaline) and cortisol released during periods of stress increase blood pressure by narrowing your blood vessels and increasing your heart rate.

The increase in blood pressure caused by stress varies, depending on your level of stress and how your body copes with stress. In some people, stress causes only a small increase in blood pressure. In others, stress can produce extreme jumps in blood pressure.

Although the effects of stress are usually only temporary, if you experience stress regularly, the increases in blood pressure it produces can over time damage your arteries, heart, brain, kidneys and eyes—just as with persistent high blood pressure.

Strategies for relieving stress

It's one thing to be aware of stress in your daily life, but it's another to know what to do about it. Here are ways you can avoid and better cope with stress.

Lifestyle changes
Making some changes in your normal routine can lessen your stress load. They include:

Get organized. Keep a written schedule of your daily activities so you're not faced with conflicts or last-minute rushes to get to an appointment or activity on time.

Simplify your schedule. Try to adopt a more relaxed pace. Set aside your "can-do" mentality and learn how to say "no" to added

> **Stress and your overall health**
>
> Stress is thought to play a role in several illnesses—both existing and new.
>
> When your heart rate increases, you become at greater risk for the development of chest pain (angina) and irregularities in your heart rhythm (arrhythmia). Surges in your heart rate and blood pressure can also trigger a heart attack or damage your heart muscle or coronary arteries. The blood-clotting chemical fibrin released when you're under stress also puts you at increased risk for formation of blood clots.
>
> The hormone cortisol released during stress may suppress your immune system, making you more susceptible to infectious diseases. Studies suggest that bacterial infections, such as tuberculosis and "strep" (streptococcus), increase with stress. So do upper respiratory viral infections such as cold or flu.
>
> Stress also can trigger headaches and may worsen asthma and intestinal problems.

responsibilities that you don't feel up to tackling. Ask others to lend a hand.

Exercise. In addition to helping control your blood pressure, exercise also helps burn off the nervous energy that stress produces. Exercise for at least 30 minutes most days of the week.

Eat well. A varied diet provides the right mix of nutrients that can help keep your immune system and other body systems working well. A healthful diet emphasizes grains, fruits, vegetables and low-fat dairy products.

Get plenty of sleep. When you're refreshed, you're better able to tackle the next day's problems. Going to sleep and awakening at a consistent time each day can help you sleep well. A bedtime ritual, such as a warm bath, reading or a snack, also helps many people relax.

Improve your appearance. Get a haircut, manicure or new outfit. Looking better will make you feel better.

Give yourself an occasional break. Get away from your regular routine and the stresses in your life. Take a vacation, even if it's just for a weekend—and plan it so you leave your stressful problems behind.

Take time to see a movie or enjoy a relaxing meal out. During the workday, take short breaks to stretch, walk, breathe deeply and relax.

Maintain good social relationships. Friends and family not only provide a release valve that lets you vent your frustrations, they also can give you helpful advice that points you toward solutions. However, avoid talking with friends and family members who tend to be negative about everything and who foster bad feelings.

Practice positive thinking. Use positive "self-talk" to tone down your critical or negative feelings. Self-talk refers to all of the things that you say to yourself—all of the thoughts that run through your head. For example, instead of "I should never make a mistake," tell yourself "I'll try to be more careful next time." This approach creates less intense negative feelings. Also try to practice old adages such as "Look for the silver lining in every cloud" and "Don't make mountains out of molehills."

Schedule worry time. Setting aside time for problem solving can keep your worries from adding up. Devote a half-hour each day to work on solutions to problems. If a worry crops up outside of "worry time," write it down and worry about it later.

Look for humor. Laughter is an inner upper. It releases chemicals in your brain that ease pain and enhance a feeling of well-being. Laughter also stimulates your heart, lungs and muscles. Just 20 seconds of laughter produces an oxygen exchange that equals about 3 minutes of aerobic exercise. Find a movie that makes you laugh out loud and books by cartoonists and comedy writers you enjoy.

Relaxation techniques

Not all stress is avoidable. There are certain events in life that you can't prevent, such as getting stuck in an unexpected traffic jam. But you can reduce the emotional and physical toll these events can cause.

When you're feeling stressed, take a few minutes to relax your body and clear your head. The following exercises are designed to help you do this. However, keep in mind that relaxation doesn't happen automatically. To develop this skill, you need to practice it daily.

Deep breathing. Unlike children, most adults breathe from their chest. Each time you breathe in your chest expands, and each time you breathe out it contracts. Children, however, generally breathe from their diaphragm, the muscle that separates the chest from the abdomen.

Deep breathing from your diaphragm—which adults can relearn—is relaxing. It also exchanges more carbon dioxide for oxygen, to give you more energy (see "Taking a breather").

Muscle tension exercises. When tension mounts, it can tighten your muscles, especially in your shoulders. To relieve the tightness, roll your shoulders, raising them toward your ears. Then relax your shoulders.

Taking a breather

Here's an exercise to help you practice deep, relaxed breathing.

1. Wear comfortable clothes that are loose around your waist. Lie on your back on a bed, a recliner chair or a padded floor. You also can sit in a chair if you prefer.

2. Place your feet slightly apart. Rest one hand on your abdomen near your navel. Put your other hand on your chest. If you're sitting, place your feet flat on the floor, relax your shoulders and place your hands in your lap or at your side.

3. Inhale through your nose, if you can, because this filters and warms the air. Exhale through your mouth.

4. Concentrate on your breathing for a few minutes and notice which hand is rising with each breath.

5. Gently exhale most of the air in your lungs.

6. Inhale while slowly counting to 4, about 1 second per count. As you inhale, slightly raise your abdomen about an inch (2.5 centimeters). You should be able to feel the movement with your hand. Don't move your chest or pull your shoulders up.

7. As you breathe in, imagine the air flowing to all parts of your body, supplying you with cleansing and energizing oxygen.

8. Pause for a second with the air in your lungs. Then slowly exhale, again counting to 4. You'll feel your abdomen slowly fall as your diaphragm relaxes. Imagine the tension flowing out of you.

9. Pause for a moment. Then begin again and repeat this exercise for 1 to 2 minutes, until you feel better. If you experience light-headedness, shorten the length or depth of your breathing.

To reduce neck tension, move your head gently in a circle going clockwise, then counterclockwise. To relieve tension in your back and torso, reach toward the ceiling and do side bends. For foot and leg tension, draw circles in the air with your feet while flexing your toes.

Daily stretching exercises also help reduce muscle tension.

Guided imagery. Also known as visualization, this method of relaxation involves lying quietly and picturing yourself in a pleasant and peaceful setting. You experience the setting with all of your senses, as if you were actually there. Imagine the sounds, scents, warmth, breezes and colors of this comforting place. The messages your brain receives as you experience these senses help your body to relax.

Meditation. It involves sitting in a comfortable position and repeating a sound or word for 20 minutes, usually twice a day. Your goal is to clear your mind of all distracting thoughts and reach a restful state.

Biofeedback. This technique helps you control body functions that you normally can't—such as your heart rate, rate of breathing, skin temperature and even your blood pressure.

Biofeedback requires the assistance of a certified biofeedback therapist and usually several training sessions. Electrodes that monitor body functions are attached to your skin, and a device, such as a beeper or a flashing light, alerts you when a certain function is beyond your target range. Then, using relaxation exercises or other strategies, you learn how to change the function until it's within your target range.

Professional help

Sometimes life's stresses can pile up and become more than you can deal with on your own. When they do, consider getting help from your doctor, a community health organization or spiritual leader. Many people believe that seeking outside help is a sign of weakness. Nothing could be further from the truth. It takes strength of character to admit you need help.

Learning how to control your stress won't guarantee you a relaxed life, good health and normal blood pressure. Unexpected problems will still occur. But having the tools to deal with stress can make those problems easier to overcome—and your blood pressure easier to control.

A sample lesson in relaxation

This stress reliever involves blocking out the world and concentrating specifically on relaxing your body.

1. Sit or lie in a comfortable position and close your eyes. Allow your jaw to drop and your eyelids to become relaxed and heavy but not tightly closed.

2. Mentally scan your body. Start with your toes and work slowly up to your legs, buttocks, torso, arms, hands, fingers, neck, head and face. As you do this, tighten each set of muscles and hold them for a count of 5 before relaxing. As the muscles relax, imagine the tension melting away.

3. During this exercise, thoughts will flow through your mind. Let them come and go without dwelling on any of them.

4. Many people find that autosuggestion, or mind over matter, helps. Suggest to yourself that you're relaxed and calm, that your hands are heavy and warm (or cool if you're hot), that your heart is beating calmly and that you're at perfect peace.

5. Breathe slowly, regularly and deeply during the exercise.

6. Once you're relaxed, imagine you're in a favorite place or in a spot of great beauty and stillness.

7. After 5 to 10 minutes, gradually rouse yourself.

Wrap-up

Key points to remember from this chapter:
- Stress can increase your blood pressure temporarily and aggravate existing high blood pressure.
- Over time, the physical effects of stress can be damaging to your health.
- Although reducing stress may not lower your blood pressure, it can make your blood pressure easier to control.
- Lifestyle changes, relaxation techniques and professional help can help you avoid or better manage stress.

Chapter 10

Medications and How They Work*

The best and safest way to control your blood pressure is through changes in your lifestyle. Sometimes, though, lifestyle changes can't reduce your blood pressure enough. To reach a desirable blood pressure, you may need the help of medication.

Medication is also often necessary if you have severe high blood pressure that needs to be reduced more quickly than lifestyle changes can accomplish, or if you have an accompanying medical condition.

Blood pressure medications, known as antihypertensives, are one of the major success stories in modern medicine. They're quite effective, and most people aren't bothered by their side effects. These drugs can control your high blood pressure and allow you to live normally with your condition. They also reduce your risk for future health problems.

There are many different types of blood pressure medication. Each lowers blood pressure in a different manner. If one medication doesn't decrease your blood pressure to a safe level, your doctor may substitute a different type or add another drug to what you're already taking. A combination of two or more low-dose drugs can lower blood pressure equally as well as one drug. In addition, drug combinations often produce fewer side effects.

The important thing is that you work with your doctor to develop a treatment plan that works for you. This approach may require patience. Finding the right medication—or combination of medications—can sometimes take time.

---

*Most drugs mentioned in the book are available in the Indian subcontinent. The brand names under which these are sold are on pages 182-84.

The different types

The major classes of medication used to control high blood pressure include:
- Diuretics
- Beta blockers
- Angiotensin-converting enzyme (ACE) inhibitors
- Angiotensin II receptor blockers
- Calcium antagonists (also known as calcium channel blockers)
- Alpha blockers
- Central-acting agents
- Direct vasodilators

Diuretics

These drugs were first introduced in the 1950s, and they're still one of the most commonly used medications to lower blood pressure. Diuretics have two major advantages. They've proven their effectiveness over the years. They're also the least expensive of all the blood pressure drugs.

Commonly referred to as fluid or water pills, diuretics reduce the volume of fluid in your body. They cause your kidneys to excrete more sodium in your urine than they would normally. The sodium takes with it water from your blood. This effect means there's a smaller volume of blood pushing through your arteries and, consequently, less pressure on your artery walls.

Diuretics are often the first drug of choice for people with stage 1 high blood pressure. They're highly effective in blacks and older adults, who more frequently are sodium-sensitive. In addition, they're commonly used in combination with other medications.

If you take a diuretic, it's important that you also limit sodium. Reducing sodium will help the drug work more effectively and with fewer side effects.

Types of diuretics

There are three classes of diuretics. Each works by affecting different parts of your kidneys. They include:

Thiazides. These are the most frequently used diuretics. They include:
- bendroflumethiazide (Naturetin)
- chlorothiazide (Diuril)
- chlorthalidone (Hygroton, Thalitone)

- hydrochlorothiazide (Esidrix, Hydrodiuril, Microzide, Oretic)
- indapamide (Lozol)
- methyclothiazide (Aquatensen, Enduron)
- metolazone (Diulo, Mykrox, Zaroxolyn)

Loop. These diuretics are more powerful than thiazides, removing a larger percentage of sodium from your kidneys. Your doctor may recommend a loop diuretic if thiazides aren't effective or if you have other conditions, such as heart or kidney failure, that also cause your body to retain fluid.

Loop diuretics include:
- bumetanide (Bumex)
- ethacrynic acid (Edecrin)
- furosemide (Lasix)
- torsemide (Demadex)

Potassium-sparing. In addition to removing sodium from your blood, diuretics remove potassium. Potassium-sparing diuretics help your body retain needed potassium. These drugs are used mainly in combination with thiazides or loop diuretics because they aren't as powerful as the others.

Potassium-sparing diuretics include:
- amiloride (Midamor)
- spironolactone (Aldactone)
- triamterene (Dyrenium)

Side effects and cautions

The leading side effect associated with diuretics is increased urination. Thiazide and loop diuretics also can cause potassium loss. That's why the two are often used in combination with a potassium-sparing diuretic.

In older adults, thiazide diuretics may cause weakness or dizziness on standing. The drugs also can cause impotence in some men, although this is uncommon. Stopping use of your medication usually causes these problems to disappear. But don't do so without your doctor's advice and guidance.

In addition, high doses of thiazide diuretics can slightly increase your blood sugar and total blood cholesterol levels. They also can increase the level of uric acid in your cells. In rare cases, this can lead to development of gout, a joint disorder.

Loop diuretics sometimes can lead to dehydration. Potassium-sparing diuretics can raise your potassium level too much. If you have kidney disease, you shouldn't take a potassium-sparing diuretic because it may cause heart rhythm irregularities and other problems from excessive potassium.

Beta blockers

Like diuretics, beta blockers have been used for many years and are often a drug of first choice for reducing blood pressure.

These drugs were originally developed to treat coronary artery disease and were later approved for treatment of high blood pressure after studies found a decrease in blood pressure among people taking them. They're also used to treat glaucoma, migraines and some tremors.

Beta blockers lower blood pressure by blocking the effects of the hormone norepinephrine (NOR-ep-i-NEF-rin), also known as noradrenaline (NOR-uh-DREN-uh-lin), which causes your heart to beat faster and your blood vessels to constrict. They also slow your kidneys' release of the enzyme renin. Renin is involved in the production of angiotensin (AN-jee-oh-TEN-sin) II, another substance that narrows your blood vessels, increasing your blood pressure.

Beta blockers successfully lower blood pressure in about half of people who try them. They're especially helpful if your high blood pressure is accompanied by certain cardiovascular conditions, such as chest pain (angina), an irregular heart rhythm (arrhythmia) or a previous heart attack. Beta blockers help control these conditions and reduce your risk for a second heart attack.

Types of beta blockers

If you have liver or kidney problems, your choice of a beta blocker may be more limited. Some beta blockers are broken down (metabolized) in your liver, others in your kidneys and some in both. If, for example, your kidneys aren't functioning properly, a drug that's metabolized in your kidneys won't work effectively.

Beta blockers also are divided according to whether they affect primarily your heart (cardioselective) or your heart and your blood vessels equally (noncardioselective). Cardioselective types generally produce fewer side effects, but they aren't recommended if you have a weakened heart muscle caused by heart failure.

Beta blockers include:
- acebutolol (Sectral)
- atenolol (Tenormin)

- betaxolol (Kerlone)
- bisoprolol (Zebeta)
- carteolol (Cartrol)
- carvedilol (Coreg)*
- labetalol (Normodyne, Trandate)*
- metoprolol (Lopressor, Toprol XL)
- nadolol (Corgard)
- penbutolol (Levatol)
- pindolol (Visken)
- propranolol (Inderal, Inderal LA)
- timolol (Blocadren)

*Combination of a beta blocker and an alpha blocker.

Side effects and cautions

Beta blockers have more frequent side effects than other blood pressure medications. However, many people who take the drugs are bothered only minimally, if at all.

Two of the most notable side effects are fatigue and a reduced capacity for strenuous physical activities. Other side effects may include cold hands, trouble sleeping, impotence, loss of sex drive, a slight increase in your blood triglyceride level and a slight decrease in your "good" (high-density lipoprotein, or HDL) blood cholesterol level.

Beta blockers aren't the best choice if you're an active young person or a serious athlete because they can limit your ability to be physically active. The drugs also aren't recommended if you have asthma or severe blockage in the conducting system of your heart (bundle branch block).

ACE inhibitors

Angiotensin-converting enzyme (ACE) inhibitors are becoming a more frequent choice among doctors for treating high blood pressure. The drugs don't have the track record of diuretics or beta blockers, but so far they've been found effective and they produce few side effects. Among blacks, ACE inhibitors are most effective when they're combined with a diuretic.

These drugs work by preventing your body from producing a substance called angiotensin I. Angiotensin I isn't harmful, but when it turns into angiotensin II it narrows your blood vessels, increasing your blood pressure. Limiting production of angiotensin also allows another substance called bradykinin (BRAD-e-KI-nin)—which keeps your vessels widened—to remain in your vessels.

ACE inhibitors include:
- benazepril (Lotensin)
- captopril (Capoten)
- enalapril (Vasotec)
- fosinopril (Monopril)
- lisinopril (Prinivil, Zestril)
- moexipril (Univasc)
- quinapril (Accupril)
- ramipril (Altace)
- trandolapril (Mavik)

Side effects and cautions

ACE inhibitors generally cause few side effects but about 20 percent of people who take them develop a dry cough. This occurs more commonly in women than in men. In some people, the cough can be persistent and annoying enough to warrant switching to another medication.

Other possible side effects may include rash, an altered sense of taste and a reduced appetite. You shouldn't take an ACE inhibitor if you have severe kidney disease because it can contribute to kidney failure. ACE inhibitors also aren't recommended if you're pregnant or plan to become pregnant. They can cause serious birth defects to the unborn child.

Angiotensin II receptor blockers

These are some of the newest drugs to be approved for treatment of high blood pressure. As their name suggests, angiotensin II receptor blockers block the action of angiotensin II, compared with ACE inhibitors, which block the formation of angiotensin I. Angiotensin II receptor blockers are also different in that they don't increase bradykinin.

These newer drugs are about equally as effective as ACE inhibitors. They also provide an extra benefit: They don't produce a dry cough.

Only a couple of angiotensin II receptor blockers are currently available. Additional brands are expected to receive Food and Drug Administration approval in the near future. Those drugs now on the market include:
- irbesartan (Avapro)
- losartan potassium (Cozaar)
- valsartan (Diovan)

Side effects and cautions
Side effects are uncommon, but in some people the drugs can cause dizziness, nasal congestion, back and leg pain, diarrhea, indigestion and insomnia.

Like ACE inhibitors, these drugs shouldn't be taken if you have severe kidney disease, you're pregnant or you're contemplating pregnancy.

Calcium antagonists

These drugs are also effective and generally well tolerated. But they're typically not a first treatment choice because some could possibly increase your risk for other serious health problems.

Calcium antagonists work by affecting the muscle cells around your arteries. These muscle cells contain tiny passages in their membranes called calcium channels. When calcium flows into them, your muscle cells contract and your arteries narrow. Calcium antagonists fill these channels—just like plugs in drains—and prevent calcium from getting into your muscle cells. The drugs don't, however, affect calcium used in the building of bone.

Some calcium antagonists have an added benefit: They slow your heart rate, potentially reducing your blood pressure even further.

Types of calcium antagonists
There are two types of calcium antagonists:

Short-acting. These drugs lower your blood pressure quickly, often in a mere half hour. But their effects last only a few hours.

Short-acting calcium antagonists aren't recommended for treating high blood pressure because they require that you take them three or four times a day. This generally results in poorer control of your blood pressure. Some studies also have linked the drugs to increased risk for heart attack, sudden cardiac death and cancer.

Long-acting. These drugs are absorbed into your body more gradually. Although it takes them longer to lower your blood pressure, they control it for a longer period.

Large randomized trials are under way to determine the safety and effectiveness of long-acting calcium antagonists. The results, which should be available within the next several years, will determine whether these drugs pose an increased risk for the same health problems linked to the short-acting type. Initial results indicate they don't.

Long-acting calcium antagonists include:
- amlodipine (Norvasc)
- diltiazem (Cardizem CD, Cardizem SR, Dilacor XR, Tiazac)*
- felodipine (Plendil)
- isradipine (DynaCirc, DynaCirc CR)
- nicardipine (Cardene SR)
- nifedipine (Adalat CC, Procardia XL)
- verapamil (Calan SR, Covera HS, Isoptin SR, Verelan)*

*These drugs also slow your heart rate.

Side effects and cautions

Possible side effects include constipation, headache, a rapid heartbeat, rash, swelling in your feet and lower legs and swelling of your gums.

You shouldn't take felodipine, nifedipine and verapamil with grapefruit juice or drink grapefruit juice 2 hours before or after taking the pills. A substance in the juice seems to reduce your liver's ability to eliminate these calcium antagonists from your body, allowing the drugs to build up and become toxic.

Alpha blockers

Alpha blockers lower your blood pressure by preventing your body's nervous system from stimulating the muscles in the walls of your smaller arteries. As a result, the muscles don't narrow (constrict) as much. Alpha blockers also reduce the effects of the hormones norepinephrine (noradrenaline) and epinephrine (adrenaline), which narrow blood vessels.

Another benefit of these drugs is that they modestly lower total blood cholesterol and triglyceride levels. If you're at risk for a heart attack because of both high blood pressure and high cholesterol, alpha blockers offer a double benefit. For older men with prostate problems, alpha blockers improve urine flow and reduce awakenings at night to go to the bathroom. Alpha blockers are also a good choice for young or physically active people who aren't good candidates for beta blockers because of their side effects.

Alpha blockers are available in both short-acting and long-acting forms. They include:
- doxazosin (Cardura), a long-acting drug
- prazosin (Minipress), a short-acting drug
- terazosin (Hytrin), a long-acting drug

Side effects and cautions

These drugs are generally well tolerated. However, when you're first prescribed the drug or if you're older, it can cause you to feel dizzy or actually faint when you stand up. That's because alpha blockers slow the time it takes your body to respond to the natural change in blood pressure when you move from a sitting or lying position to a standing position.

To reduce this problem, your doctor may prescribe only a small initial dose of the drug and instruct you to take it before you go to bed at night. After you've adapted to the drug, your doctor will slowly increase the dosage. It's best to take alpha blockers at bedtime, unless your doctor prescribes otherwise.

Other possible side effects include a headache, a pounding heartbeat, nausea and weakness. Over time, the medications also can lose their effectiveness. However, the addition of a diuretic can prevent this.

Central-acting agents

Unlike other blood pressure medications that work on your blood vessels, central-acting agents work on your brain. They prevent your brain from sending signals to your nervous system to speed up your heart rate and narrow your blood vessels.

These medications, also called central adrenergic (AD-ren-UR-jik) inhibitors, aren't used as often as they once were because they can produce strong side effects. However, they're still prescribed in certain circumstances. Your doctor may recommend a central-acting agent if you're prone to panic attacks, you have incidents of low blood sugar or you're going through alcohol or drug withdrawal. The drugs can help reduce symptoms of these conditions.

One type of central-acting agent, clonidine, is available as a skin patch. This is helpful if you have trouble taking oral medication. Another type of central-acting agent, methyldopa, is often recommended to pregnant women with high blood pressure who can't take other blood pressure drugs because of risks to themselves and the baby.

Central-acting agents include:
- clonidine (Catapres)
- guanabenz (Wytensin)
- guanadrel (Hylorel)
- guanethidine (Ismelin)
- guanfacine (Tenex)

- methyldopa (Aldomet)
- reserpine (Serpasil)

Side effects and cautions
These drugs can produce extreme fatigue, drowsiness or sedation. They also can cause impotence, dry mouth, headaches, weight gain, impaired thinking and psychological problems, including depression.

Stopping use of some central-acting agents can cause your blood pressure to increase to dangerously high levels very quickly. If you're bothered by side effects and want to quit taking your drug, see your doctor and develop a plan for gradually stopping its use.

Direct vasodilators

These potent medications are used mainly to treat difficult cases of high blood pressure that don't respond well to other medications. They work directly on the muscles in the walls of your arteries, preventing the muscles from tightening and your arteries from narrowing.

Direct vasodilators include:
- hydralazine (Apresoline)
- minoxidil (Loniten)

Side effects and cautions
Common side effects of direct vasodilators include a fast heartbeat and retention of water—neither of which is very desirable if you have high blood pressure. That's why doctors typically prescribe direct vasodilators with a beta blocker and a diuretic, which can reduce these symptoms.

Other side effects may include gastrointestinal problems, dizziness, headaches, nasal congestion, excessive hair growth all over your body and swelling of your gums. Hydralazine taken in large doses can increase your risk for lupus, a connective tissue disease.

Emergency medications

If your blood pressure reaches a dangerously high level, it may be necessary to reduce it rapidly to avoid serious damage to your organs, and even death. Examples of these situations include a heart attack, heart failure, stroke, sudden blindness or a rupture in the wall of your aorta.

During blood pressure emergencies, doctors inject high blood pressure medication into your veins. The goal is to lower your blood pressure by 25 percent within several minutes to 2 hours. Reducing your blood pressure too fast can cause other serious, even fatal, conditions. Once your blood pressure is reduced 25 percent, then the goal is to lower your blood pressure to near 160/100 mm Hg within 6 hours.

The types of injectable medications used in hypertensive emergencies include:
- Vasodilators, such as fenoldopam, nicardipine hydrochloride, nitroglycerin and sodium nitroprusside
- Alpha and beta blockers, such as esmolol hydrochloride, labetalol hydrochloride and phentolamine

Combination drug therapy

Approximately half of people with stage 1 or 2 high blood pressure can control their blood pressure with just one drug. If one drug isn't effective, your doctor may increase the dosage, provided you aren't experiencing significant side effects. Other options are to try a different drug or add another drug to the one you're already taking.

Combination drug therapy is quite common and beneficial. By using a combination of two or more drugs, doctors can increase from 50 percent to 80 percent the number of people who respond positively to high blood pressure medication. An advantage of combination therapy is that you generally take smaller doses of each drug. This reduces your risk for side effects from your medication.

When using combination therapy, your doctor looks for medications that enhance each other's effectiveness or reduce each other's side effects. A diuretic, for example, can enhance the effectiveness of beta blockers, ACE inhibitors and angiotensin II receptor antagonists (see "Working in combination," on the following page).

Finding the right medication

Your goal should be to find a drug or combination of drugs that reduces your blood pressure to a normal level without unbearable side effects. Almost all people taking blood pressure medication are eventually able to come up with a drug regimen that allows them to feel well and be fully active, and that also produces few, if any, side effects.

In addition to the effectiveness of a drug, your doctor will consider these factors in determining what's the right medication for you:

Your tolerance to the drug. If taking a certain medication produces side effects that are unpleasant to live with, such as impotence, headaches or fatigue, then it's probably not the best drug for you.

Working in combination

It's common for two drugs to be mixed together into the same tablet or capsule. Some examples of high blood pressure medications in which two drugs are combined into one are listed here.

Combinations of a diuretic and beta blocker:
- bendroflumethiazide and nadolol (Corzide)
- chlorthalidone and atenolol (Tenoretic)
- hydrochlorothiazide and bisoprolol (Ziac)
- hydrochlorothiazide and propranolol (Inderide LA)
- hydrochlorothiazide and metoprolol (Lopressor HCT)

Combinations of a diuretic and an ACE inhibitor:
- hydrochlorothiazide and benazepril (Lotensin HCT)
- hydrochlorothiazide and captopril (Capozide)
- hydrochlorothiazide and enalapril (Vaseretic)
- hydrochlorothiazide and lisinopril (Prinzide, Zestoretic)

Combinations of a diuretic and an angiotensin II receptor antagonist:
- hydrochlorothiazide and losartan potassium (Hyzaar)
- hydrochlorothiazide and valsartan (Diovan HCT)

Combinations of two diuretics:
- amiloride and hydrochlorothiazide (Moduretic)
- spironolactone and hydrochlorothiazide (Aldactazide)
- triamterene and hydrochlorothiazide (Dyazide, Maxzide)

Combinations of a calcium antagonist and an ACE inhibitor:
- amlodipine and benazepril (Lotrel)
- diltiazem and enalapril (Teczem)
- verapamil and trandolapril (Tarka)
- felodipine and enalapril (Lexxel)

In fact, the medication's side effects may seem worse to live with than your high blood pressure, which produces no apparent symptoms. But don't stop taking the medication on your own. Talk to your doctor.

Your compliance with the prescription. If a certain medication is fairly complicated to take and you have a busy schedule, it's possible you may forget to take it. Because it's vital that you take your medication properly, the medication your doctor prescribes should fit your lifestyle.

Your ability to pay for the medication. Some people don't have insurance or financial resources to pay for their drugs. A drug doesn't do you any good if you can't take it correctly because you can't afford it.

A look ahead

Even with the wide variety of blood pressure drugs currently in use, researchers and drug companies continue to seek new medications that are more effective and produce even fewer side effects.

Drug research

Some new drugs being studied include:

Dual metalloprotease inhibitors. They block a substance that narrows your arteries and increase another that opens them wider. Researchers believe these drugs could be even more effective than ACE inhibitors, reducing blood pressure in up to 80 percent of people with high blood pressure.

Endothelin inhibitors. The drugs prevent a powerful blood vessel constrictor called ET-1 from getting into the muscles in the walls of your blood vessels.

Natriuretic peptide clearance inhibitors. They help ensure that certain compounds that fight high blood pressure remain in your body.

Renin inhibitors. The drugs block development of the enzyme renin, needed to produce angiotensin II, a powerful blood

> **For more information on medications, visit Mayo Clinic Health Oasis**
> Medications for high blood pressure are continually being developed and marketed. For information on new drugs or to learn more about existing medications, visit our Web site at *www.mayohealth.org*.

Vasopressin antagonists. This type of drug prevents blood vessel narrowing linked to the retention of sodium. If approved, the drug could be particularly useful for people who are sodium-sensitive.

Gene research

In 95 percent of people with high blood pressure, the specific cause of their condition is unknown. Some of the research being done on high blood pressure involves identifying genes that may trigger the disease.

Initial research indicates that high blood pressure is a complex illness that doesn't follow the classic rules of inheritance. Instead of stemming from a single defective gene, it appears to be a multifaceted disorder that involves interaction between several genes. In addition, environmental factors, including weight, sodium use and physical activity, also appear to play a role in gene interaction.

However, if gene research is successful, the results could one day lead to development of new drugs that prevent high blood pressure by controlling specific genes.

Wrap-up

Key points to remember from this chapter:
- You may need medication if lifestyle changes aren't effective, you have severe high blood pressure or you have another medical condition that could benefit from drug use.
- Half of people with high blood pressure needing medication can control their blood pressure with just one drug. Others need a combination of two or three drugs.
- A diuretic or a beta blocker is often prescribed for uncomplicated high blood pressure because of their successful track records.
- Most people taking blood pressure medication are bothered only minimally by side effects.
- Finding the right drug or combination of drugs to control your blood pressure may require time and patience.

Chapter 11

Special Concerns

High blood pressure most often develops between the ages of 30 and 60, but it has no boundaries. It can affect anyone at any time. Your blood pressure also is influenced by your sex, race and other medical conditions. When determining the best way to treat or prevent high blood pressure, all of these factors must be considered.

This chapter looks at factors unique to women, management of high blood pressure among specific populations and groups, treatment of difficult-to-control high blood pressure and what to do in a hypertensive emergency.

Issues for women

Previous studies on the development and treatment of high blood pressure have primarily involved men. Yet, approximately 60 percent of all people diagnosed with high blood pressure are women.

As it becomes apparent that women may respond differently to medication and that they often develop the disease for different reasons and at different times in their lives, more studies are now focusing specifically on issues that affect women.

Oral contraceptives

Oral contraceptives ("the pill") are a common form of birth control. They contain small amounts of the hormones estrogen and progestin that prevent pregnancy.

When oral contraceptives first came on the market decades ago, they contained much larger doses of estrogen and progestin than they do now. Back then, about 5 percent of all women who took oral contraceptives developed high blood pressure. Today, the hormone dose in oral contraceptives is about 80 percent less than that in earlier versions, and high blood pressure from oral contraceptives is rare. The drugs may cause your systolic blood pressure to increase slightly, but the increase is usually so small that it's nothing to worry about.

If you're among the few women whose blood pressure does increase significantly with use of an oral contraceptive, your doctor may recommend that you stop taking the pill. Within a few months, your blood pressure should return to normal. If alternative birth control isn't possible and you want to continue taking the pill, you'll need to take steps to lower your blood pressure through lifestyle changes and, possibly, medication.

Pregnancy

It's quite possible for women with high blood pressure to have a normal pregnancy and childbirth. However, if you have high blood pressure, you have a greater risk for complications during your pregnancy which can affect both you and your unborn child.

Your doctor will want to monitor your pregnancy and your blood pressure closely, especially during the last 3 months (third trimester), when complications are most likely to occur.

Uncommon, but possible, complications for the mother include swelling, heart failure, seizures, a decline in kidney or liver function, vision changes and bleeding. Possible complications for your unborn child include impairment in growth, greater risk for separation of the placenta from the uterine wall and greater risk for reduced oxygen during labor.

Talk with your doctor about possible health risks before becoming pregnant. You may want to change your medication because some blood pressure drugs shouldn't be taken during the first 3 months of pregnancy. Also, inform your doctor as soon as you become pregnant.

If you see a different doctor during your pregnancy, make sure to mention during your first visit that you have high blood pressure. Because blood pressure normally decreases during the early and middle stages of pregnancy, a doctor who's unfamiliar with your medical history may not realize you have high blood pressure.

If you have stage 2 or stage 3 high blood pressure, your doctor will likely recommend that you continue to take your medication while you're pregnant. The benefit you receive from managing your blood pressure with medication outweighs the risk of side effects to your developing baby.

If you have stage 1 high blood pressure, discuss the benefits and disadvantages of taking medication with your doctor. For milder high blood pressure, it's not clear that the benefits of continuing your medication outweigh the possible risks to your baby.

For women who need to take medication during pregnancy, the central-acting drug methyldopa (METH-ul-DO-pah) is sometimes used. Beta blockers also may be prescribed in certain situations. Angiotensin-converting enzyme (ACE) inhibitors and angiotensin II receptor blockers shouldn't be taken during pregnancy because they can potentially slow growth of the fetus, cause birth defects and possibly be fatal to the unborn infant.

Pregnancy-induced high blood pressure

A small percentage of women develop high blood pressure during their pregnancy. This condition is sometimes referred to as gestational hypertension. It most often happens during the later stages of pregnancy, and in most cases the increase is mild. Once the pregnancy is complete, blood pressure returns to normal.

If you develop pregnancy-induced high blood pressure—especially if you have stage 1 high blood pressure—medication generally isn't necessary. But you may need to limit sodium and follow a diet that emphasizes grains, fruits, vegetables and low-fat dairy products—foods that help control high blood pressure.

Only if your blood pressure increases a significant amount, putting your health or your baby's in jeopardy, is medication recommended.

In most cases, pregnancy-induced high blood pressure is a sign of one of two things: It's an early indicator that you're likely to develop high blood pressure later in life or it's an early warning to a condition called preeclampsia.

Preeclampsia

Preeclampsia (PREE-e-KLAMP-see-ah) occurs in about 25 percent of women who develop pregnancy-induced high blood pressure—typically after the 20th week of pregnancy. It's characterized by high blood pressure, swelling of your hands and face and a large amount of protein in your urine. Left untreated, it can lead to serious, even deadly, complications.

At one time, preeclampsia was called toxemia because it was thought to result from a toxin in your bloodstream. Doctors now know that a toxin isn't responsible. However, the exact cause of preeclampsia is unknown. Certain factors, though, can increase your risk for developing preeclampsia. They include:

- A first pregnancy
- A family history of preeclampsia
- Carrying twins
- Diabetes
- Kidney problems before pregnancy
- Pregnancy in your early teens or past age 40

An important reason your blood pressure is checked at every doctor visit during your pregnancy is that women who develop preeclampsia often have no symptoms at first. By the time they do appear, the condition is often advanced. In addition to swelling and increased protein in your urine, you may also experience sudden weight gain of more than 2 pounds (0.9 kilogram) in a week or 6 pounds (2.7 kilograms) in a month. Other signs and symptoms may include headaches, vision problems and pain in your upper abdomen.

Your blood pressure and urine will be checked regularly. Your doctor also may perform blood tests to check your blood platelet count and to see how well your liver and kidneys are functioning. A low blood platelet level and increased liver enzyme values indicate a severe form of preeclampsia called HELLP (hemolysis, elevated liver enzymes, low platelet count) syndrome.

Severe preeclampsia requires you to stay in the hospital. Your health and your baby's are continuously monitored. You also may be given the drug magnesium sulfate, which increases blood flow to your uterus and helps prevent seizures. If tests indicate that your or your baby's health may be at significant risk, early delivery of your baby may be necessary. Labor may be induced or a cesarean section performed.

Mild preeclampsia often can be managed at home with bed rest. You'll be asked to lie on your left side to allow blood to flow more freely to the placenta. Your doctor will want to see you frequently to check your blood pressure and urine, do blood tests and check the status of the baby. You also may need to check your blood pressure on a regular basis at home.

After delivery, your blood pressure should return to normal within several days to several weeks. If your blood pressure is still at stage 2 or stage 3 when you leave the hospital you may need to take blood pressure medication. Most women are able to taper off the medication after a few months.

Eclampsia

Eclampsia is a life-threatening condition that can develop when symptoms of preeclampsia aren't controlled. The incidence of eclampsia is about 1 in 1,500 pregnancies.

Eclampsia can permanently damage your brain, liver or kidneys, and it can be fatal for both you and your unborn child. Symptoms of eclampsia include:
- Pain in the upper right side of your abdomen
- Severe headache and vision problems, including seeing flashing lights
- Severe convulsions
- Unconsciousness

Hormone replacement therapy

Unlike oral contraceptives—in which the hormones estrogen and progestin may slightly increase your blood pressure—in hormone replacement therapy these hormones don't increase blood pressure. According to some studies, hormone replacement therapy may even lower blood pressure a minimal amount.

The difference is related mainly to the level of estrogen. Hormone replacement therapy contains considerably lower doses of estrogen than oral contraceptives. Another reason may be that hormone replacement therapy contains different types of progestin.

Hormone replacement therapy often is prescribed to women after menopause to reduce their risk for cardiovascular disease and lessen postmenopausal symptoms, such as hot flashes and vaginal dryness. Whether you're healthy or you have high blood pressure, you can take hormone replacement therapy without worry that it will increase your blood pressure. If you've had a hysterectomy, you'll need to take only estrogen.

High blood pressure in children

Infants are born with a low blood pressure that increases quickly during the first month of life. During childhood, your blood pressure continues to slowly increase until you reach your teens, when it reaches a level similar to that in an adult.

Blood pressure generally isn't measured in infants and young children because getting an accurate measurement is difficult. However, once your child reaches age 3, your doctor should check his or her blood pressure at every well-child visit.

A different method is used to determine high blood pressure in children than in adults. Your child's blood pressure is rated on a percentile basis, taking into account his or her age and height. At any age, taller children tend to have higher blood pressures than children who are shorter or of average height. A blood pressure reading above the 95th percentile is considered high.

High blood pressure in children is uncommon. However, as an increasing number of children become less physically active and more obese, a greater percentage of them may run the risk of developing high blood pressure in their teens.

More often than in adults, high blood pressure in children indicates that something else is wrong and the increase in blood pressure is a symptom of that condition. For that reason, your doctor likely will perform several tests to find the reason for your child's increased blood pressure. If all test results are normal and all other possible causes are eliminated, then it may be that your child has high blood pressure for the same reasons adults get it. Factors such as obesity, a poor diet and lack of exercise can lead to high blood pressure in children as well as in adults.

For children whose high blood pressure has no clear cause, lifestyle changes are a common treatment. It can be hard for youngsters to stick to a diet and exercise plan, especially for teenagers who want to control their own lifestyle choices. But it's important to stress these changes as being very important to your child's future health. High blood pressure in children that's ignored or not controlled can lead to heart or vision problems.

Your doctor may prescribe medication if your child's blood pressure is quite high or if lifestyle changes aren't working. The same medications used to control high blood pressure in adults are used for children, only in smaller doses. In some specific situations, high blood pressure in children may be cured by surgery.

High blood pressure in older adults

There was a time when high blood pressure in older adults was ignored because it wasn't thought to be a problem. However, recent studies have shown that no matter what your age, controlling high blood pressure can reduce your risk for stroke or heart attack—and possibly add years to your life.

With age, your diastolic blood pressure decreases slightly, but your systolic blood pressure often increases. That's because your blood vessels become more rigid as you get older, causing your heart to work harder to pump blood throughout your body. The vessels simply can't stretch to accommodate the same amount of blood, so the pressure on your artery walls becomes greater.

If your systolic pressure increases to 160 mm Hg or more while your diastolic measurement stays normal, then you may have a condition called isolated systolic hypertension (ISH). About half of older adults with high blood pressure have this condition.

Doctors were once reluctant to treat isolated systolic hypertension because they thought it was a normal result of aging. However, a 5-year study shows that treating this form of high blood pressure can prevent 24,000 strokes and 50,000 severe cardiovascular problems, including heart attack, each year. Another study from Europe found a 40 percent reduction in strokes among people being treated for isolated systolic hypertension.

Losing weight if you're overweight and walking daily to stay active can help reduce your blood pressure. Because you may become more sodium-sensitive with age, limiting sodium to no more than 2,400 milligrams daily also can help control high blood pressure.

If you need medication, a diuretic, a calcium antagonist or a diuretic combined with a beta blocker is often the most effective in older adults.

High blood pressure and ethnic groups

As early as 1932, researchers noted a difference in blood pressures between whites and blacks of African-American descent living in New Orleans. Blood pressures among 6,000 black males were 7 mm Hg higher than among a group of 8,000 white males.

If you're black, you're twice as likely to develop high blood pressure than if you were white. You're also more likely to develop serious complications from the disease or to die of a stroke or heart attack related to your high blood pressure. Less access to medical care is one factor. However, the difference between blacks and whites is primarily genetic.

The good news, though, is that with proper medical care, strokes and heart attacks from high blood pressure can be reduced equally as well in blacks as in whites.

The first drug of choice if you're black—and the one that's often the most effective—is a diuretic. However, because blacks tend to have more severe high blood pressure, you may need another medication in addition to a diuretic to control your condition.

Blacks aren't the only ethnic group at increased risk for high blood pressure. The prevalence of high blood pressure among some populations of American Indians is higher than in whites. People of Hispanic background have about the same incidence of high blood pressure as whites. In some areas, the incidence is slightly lower than in whites.

High blood pressure and other illnesses

Often, high blood pressure is accompanied by other medical conditions that make it more difficult to treat and control. If you have another chronic illness in addition to high blood pressure, it's especially important that you see your doctor regularly.

Cardiovascular problems

Cardiovascular conditions that often coexist with high blood pressure include:

Arrhythmia. High blood pressure can cause your heart to beat in an irregular rhythm. You're at greater risk for developing this condition if your blood contains low levels of potassium or magnesium.

To control or prevent arrhythmia, consume plenty of foods containing potassium and magnesium. If this doesn't help, your doctor may recommend that you take supplements to keep your potassium and magnesium levels normal.

Arteriosclerosis and atherosclerosis. If you have one or both of these conditions, which cause your arteries to become stiff or narrowed, your doctor may prescribe a low-dose thiazide diuretic or a beta blocker to reduce the volume or intensity of blood flowing through your arteries.

Heart failure. Heart failure causes you to develop an enlarged, weakened heart, which has a hard time pumping your blood to meet your body's needs. In some cases, this can cause fluid to build up in your lungs or your feet and legs.

An ACE inhibitor and diuretics are prescribed most often if you have heart failure in addition to high blood pressure. ACE inhibitors reduce blood pressure by dilating your blood vessels, without interfering with your heart's pumping action. Diuretics reduce fluid buildup. In some specific cases, a beta blocker may be appropriate.

Coronary artery disease. If you have high blood pressure, there's a 50 percent chance that the major arteries leading to your heart (coronary) also are damaged. Damage to these arteries increases your risk for a heart attack.

Beta blockers and ACE inhibitors are often the drugs of choice for people with high blood pressure and coronary artery disease because in addition to lowering your blood pressure, they reduce your risk for a heart attack. If you've already had a heart attack, beta blockers can reduce your risk for a second heart attack.

Diabetes

High blood pressure is nearly twice as common in people with diabetes. If you're black, your chances of having both diabetes and high blood pressure are double that of a white person. If you're Hispanic, that chance increases to three times. Although Hispanics have about the same risk for high blood pressure as whites, their risk for diabetes is much higher. Once you develop diabetes, your odds for developing high blood pressure increase.

Whatever your ethnic group, having both diabetes and high blood pressure is serious. Between 35 percent and 75 percent of all complications associated with diabetes can be attributed to having high blood pressure. High blood pressure also increases your chances for death from diabetes.

If you have diabetes and high blood pressure, your goal should be to lower your blood pressure to 130/85 mm Hg or below.

If you have type 2 diabetes—the most common type that typically develops in middle adulthood—it's important that you stop smoking if you smoke, follow a healthful diet, get regular physical activity and limit alcohol. The same lifestyle choices that lead to high blood pressure also lead to type 2 diabetes.

If you need to take blood pressure medication, ACE inhibitors or angiotensin II receptor blockers are prescribed most often. They help protect your kidneys, which are at a high risk for damage from both diseases. These drugs also have a low rate of side effects. Diuretics, beta blockers, calcium antagonists or alpha blockers also may be used.

High cholesterol

Eighty percent of people with high blood pressure also have high cholesterol. Because both high cholesterol and high blood pressure increase your risk for a heart attack and stroke, you need to work hard to lower your cholesterol level as well as your blood pressure level.

The same lifestyle changes that lower blood pressure also will lower your cholesterol. However, approximately half of people with high cholesterol need the help of cholesterol medication to reduce their cholesterol level to normal.

As for blood pressure medications, you shouldn't take high doses of thiazide and loop diuretics if you also have high cholesterol. They can increase your cholesterol level and your triglycerides, another type of blood fat. Low doses of these drugs, though, don't produce the same effects. High doses of beta blockers also aren't a good choice because they may reduce your "good" (high-density lipoprotein, or HDL) cholesterol level, as well as increase your triglyceride value. However, should you need to take high doses of either type, diet and cholesterol medication can help counteract the cholesterol increase.

Medications most often recommended if you have high blood pressure and high cholesterol are ACE inhibitors, angiotensin II receptor blockers, alpha blockers, calcium antagonists and central-acting agents.

Kidney disease

High blood pressure can lead to chronic renal failure, a condition in which your kidneys no longer function. If you have kidney disease, it's important to prevent further damage to your kidneys as a result of your high blood pressure.

Kidney failure is especially a concern if you're black. Blacks are nearly four times as likely to have end-stage renal disease, which leads to irreversible kidney failure and, ultimately, death.

Your goal should be to reduce your blood pressure to below 130/85 mm Hg. Once your blood pressure is below this level, decline in your kidney function slows.

ACE inhibitors are often the best medication for preventing further damage to your kidneys. However, they aren't recommended for severe disease and they're not as effective in blacks. Among blacks, ACE inhibitors are commonly combined with a diuretic or calcium antagonist.

Difficult-to-control high blood pressure

What if you've been following your doctor's orders and taking your medication, but you still aren't able to lower your blood pressure?

It could be you're among 5 percent to 10 percent of all people with "resistant" or "refractory" high blood pressure, meaning high blood pressure that's resistant to treatment. Resistant high blood pressure is defined as blood pressure that can't be brought below 140/90 mm Hg using a combination of three different types of medication.

It's rare for medication not to lower high blood pressure. Often, it just takes time and experimentation with different drugs to find the combination of drugs that works best.

If your medication isn't working, many times the first step is to try a different type of drug. Some medications work better for some people than for others. The next step may be to add another medication to the one you're already taking, perhaps even a third drug. Medications often have more powerful effects on your blood pressure when working in concert than working alone. Rarely does anyone start out taking three different medications, but sometimes this approach may be necessary.

Often, resistant high blood pressure stems from not making necessary changes in your lifestyle. If your blood pressure isn't responding to drug therapy, ask yourself the following questions:

- *Have I been taking my medication exactly as prescribed?* You need to take your medication as your doctor ordered or it may not work. If you think the pills cost too much, or you find the regimen too hard to follow, talk to your doctor. Less expensive medications or drugs that you take only once a day often can be found. It's also important that you tell your doctor about all the drugs you take, including over-the-counter products. They could be interfering with your blood pressure medication.
- *Have I cut down on sodium?* Remember, this doesn't mean table salt alone. Even if you aren't salting your foods, you may be eating processed foods with too much sodium.

- *Am I drinking too much alcohol?* Alcohol can keep your blood pressure increased, especially if you consume large amounts during short intervals. Your medication may not be enough to combat the effects of alcohol.
- *Have I seriously tried to quit smoking?* Like alcohol, tobacco can keep your blood pressure increased if you smoke frequently.
- *Have I gained weight?* Generally, losing weight decreases your blood pressure. A significant weight gain can increase it and make it harder to control.
- *Have I been sleeping well?* A condition called sleep apnea can increase your blood pressure. It occurs most frequently in older adults. People with sleep apnea stop breathing for short periods during the night. This stresses your heart and can increase your blood pressure. Treating the condition can reduce your blood pressure.

> **Are your readings misleading?**
> In rare cases, resistant high blood pressure may be the result of a mistake in your diagnosis. Two conditions can make your blood pressure appear higher than it actually is. They are:
> - Pseudohypertension
> - "White-coat" hypertension
>
> See Chapter 3 (pages 39 and 41) for more on these conditions.

If you, along with your doctor, have exhausted these possibilities, you have a couple of options. To begin with, you need to consider stepping up positive changes to your lifestyle. If you can walk another block, lose 1 more pound or make more improvements in your diet, your high blood pressure may become less resistant to treatment.

Your other options include adding a fourth drug to your daily regimen or increasing the dosage of your current medication. The danger with each is increased risk for side effects from the medication.

High blood pressure emergencies

Throughout this book, you've read how uncontrolled high blood pressure can erode your health by wearing on your body and gradually damaging your organs. Sometimes, though, high blood pressure can suddenly become life-threatening, requiring immediate care. When this happens, it's a hypertensive emergency.

Hypertensive emergencies are rare. They occur when your blood pressure increases to a dangerously high level and is accompanied by other serious symptoms (see "Emergency warning signs"). Generally, a reading of 180/110 mm Hg or greater is considered dangerously high. However, if you have another medical condition, lower elevations in your blood pressure also can trigger a hypertensive emergency.

To prevent damage to your organs, your blood pressure needs to be lowered promptly but gradually. Lowering it too fast can interfere with normal blood flow, possibly resulting in too little blood to your heart, brain and other organs.

The simplest answer for a dangerous increase in your blood pressure is that you've forgotten to take your medication and your body is reacting to that oversight.

Other causes include:
- Stroke
- Heart attack
- Heart failure
- Kidney failure
- Rupture in your aorta
- Interaction between your blood pressure medication and another drug
- Eclampsia (see page 143)

Emergency warning signs
In addition to dangerously high blood pressure, symptoms that often signal a hypertensive emergency include:
- A severe headache, accompanied by confusion and blurred vision
- Severe chest pain
- Marked shortness of breath
- Nausea and vomiting
- Seizures
- Unresponsiveness

Don't drink or eat anything, and lie down until emergency help arrives or you get to a hospital.

Urgency vs. emergency

If at least three blood pressure measurements taken a few minutes apart produce readings of 180/110 mm Hg or higher but you aren't experiencing any other symptoms, contact your doctor or another health care professional at your doctor's office right away. If that isn't possible, go to a hospital near you.

Although a blood pressure of 180/110 mm Hg alone isn't considered an emergency, it's important that you be evaluated as soon as you can. Left untreated for more than a few hours, pressures this high could possibly lead to an emergency.

Wrap-up

Key points to remember from this chapter:
- Newer oral contraceptives and hormone replacement therapy rarely produce or worsen high blood pressure.
- High blood pressure during pregnancy needs to be monitored closely. It can be a symptom of a condition called preeclampsia. Left untreated, preeclampsia can lead to life-threatening eclampsia.
- High blood pressure in children is uncommon. More often than in adults, it may be a symptom of another health problem.
- There are benefits to treating high blood pressure at any age.
- Blacks have twice the incidence of high blood pressure and more complications from it. Some American Indian populations also have higher rates of high blood pressure.
- High blood pressure associated with diabetes, high cholesterol, cardiovascular disease or kidney disease needs aggressive treatment.
- Dangerously high blood pressure accompanied by other symptoms needs immediate treatment.

Chapter 12

Staying in Control

High blood pressure isn't an illness you can treat and then ignore. It's a condition you need to manage the rest of your life. This can sometimes be difficult because you can't feel or see anything wrong. With many diseases, such as arthritis or allergies, symptoms motivate you to seek treatment. You feel the flaring pain of arthritic joints. You experience the sneezing, itchy eyes and cough. Control comes naturally because you want these symptoms to go away.

Lack of symptoms is why people with high blood pressure often don't take steps to treat their disease and why only about one in four Americans with high blood pressure is in control of the condition.

Managing high blood pressure—measuring your blood pressure at home, taking your medications properly, making regular visits to your doctor—is essential. It can significantly increase your chances for living a longer, healthier life, despite high blood pressure.

Home monitoring

Your doctor's office isn't the only place to measure your blood pressure. You can do it yourself at home.

Blood pressure monitors are available at medical supply stores and in many pharmacies. They're not that difficult to use—especially once you've had a little practice.

Benefits of home monitoring

Measuring your blood pressure at home can help:

Track your treatment. Because high blood pressure has no symptoms, the only way to make sure lifestyle changes or your medications are working is to check your blood pressure regularly.

Promote better control. When you take the initiative to measure your own blood pressure, this responsible act tends to rub off on other areas. It can give you added incentive to eat more healthfully, increase your activity level and take your medication properly.

Identify "white-coat" hypertension. Simply going to a doctor's office can make some people nervous, increasing their blood pressures. Home monitoring can help determine whether you have true high blood pressure or white-coat hypertension.

Save money. Home monitoring saves you the cost of going to your doctor's office to have your blood pressure taken. This is especially true when you first start to take medication or your doctor adjusts your medication. In these cases, frequent measurements help ensure better control.

Types of blood pressure monitors

Not all blood pressure monitors are the same. Some are easier to use. Others are more reliable, and some are inaccurate and a waste of money.

Blood pressure monitors are available in these forms:

Mercury-column models. These monitors have long glass gauges that look like oversized thermometers. You often see them in hospitals and in doctors' offices, and for good reason. They're the most accurate—the standard by which all other monitors are judged.

Mercury-column models measure how high your blood pressure pushes the column of mercury inside the glass gauge. The advantage of mercury-column monitors is that they don't need to be adjusted (calibrated) to ensure accuracy.

But this type of monitor can be difficult to use, especially if you have trouble hearing or using your hands. Standard models require use of a stethoscope to listen for your heartbeat and a hand-operated bulb pump to inflate the blood pressure cuff. However, some mercury-column monitors come with a built-in stethoscope.

Mercury-column monitors also must rest on a flat surface during the measurement and be read at eye level.

Spring-gauge models. These monitors feature a round dial activated by a spring-pressure gauge. Each degree the needle moves in the dial is set to match a millimeter of mercury.

Health care professionals often recommend spring-gauge models because they're inexpensive and easy to transport. In addition, some gauges are extra large, for easier reading, and some models have a built-in stethoscope for easier use.

A disadvantage is that once a year you need to verify the monitor's accuracy by comparing it with a mercury-column model. You can do this by taking your monitor with you to your doctor's office. If the reading is more than 4 millimeters off, you should replace the unit.

Like mercury-column models, standard spring-gauge monitors aren't recommended if you have trouble hearing or if you have poor dexterity in your hands. They also require use of a stethoscope and bulb pump.

Electronic models. Also referred to as digital monitors, these models are the most popular and the easiest to use. They're also the most expensive. Prices can run as high as $160, compared with as little as $30 for a standard spring-gauge model.

Electronic blood pressure monitors generally require that you do just two things: Put the cuff on your arm and push a button. The cuff automatically inflates with air and then slowly deflates. Built-in sensors detect your blood pressure and display the measurement on a screen.

To get an accurate reading, place the sensor over the main artery (brachial) in your arm. It's also important that the cuff fits you properly. Have your doctor or other health care professional measure your arm and determine the appropriate size cuff for you.

Like spring-gauge models, you need to check the monitor's accuracy at least once a year. Electronic monitors are less accurate than the previous types and the easiest to damage.

If you have an irregular heart rhythm, you shouldn't use an electronic monitor because it will give you an inaccurate reading.

Finger or wrist monitors. To make blood pressure monitors more compact and easier to use, some manufacturers have produced models that easily measure blood pressure in your wrist or finger, instead of your upper arm.

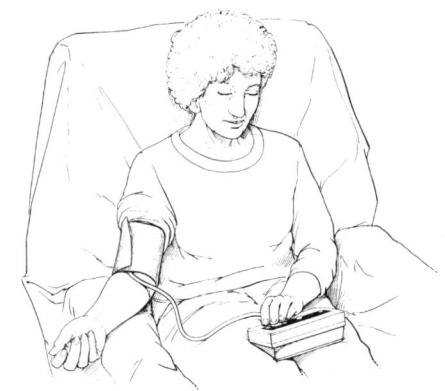

Electronic blood pressure monitors are the most popular and easiest to use. They're also the most expensive.

Unfortunately, the technology of finger monitors hasn't caught up with their simplicity of use. Avoid them because they're inaccurate. Wrist monitors are fairly accurate as long as you make sure your wrist is at the level of your heart when you take your measurement.

Home monitoring tips

Learning to take your blood pressure correctly takes practice and a little training. After you purchase a blood pressure monitor, take it with you to your doctor's office.

In addition to making sure it works properly, your doctor or other health care professional can help you learn how to use it. Some medical facilities also provide classes on how to take your blood pressure. Keep in mind that if you have an irregular heart rhythm, getting an accurate reading will be more difficult.

To accurately measure your blood pressure:
- Don't measure your blood pressure right after you get up in the morning. Wait until after you've been active for an hour or more. If you exercise right after you awaken, wait for 2 hours after exercising to measure your blood pressure. Your blood pressure decreases to a temporary low for 1 to 2 hours after exercise.
- Wait for at least a half hour after you've eaten, smoked or used caffeine or alcohol to measure your blood pressure. Food, tobacco, caffeine and alcohol can increase your pressure.
- Go to the bathroom first. A full bladder increases your blood pressure slightly.
- Sit quietly for about 5 minutes before taking a reading.
- Remember that your blood pressure varies throughout the day. Readings are often a little higher in the morning. Your mood also can affect your blood pressure. If you've had a difficult day, don't be alarmed if your blood pressure reflects it.
- Use proper technique. Follow these 10 steps when taking your blood pressure. If you have an electronic device, some steps won't apply.

1. Sit comfortably with your legs and ankles uncrossed and your back supported against the back of a chair. Rest your arm at heart level on a table or the arm of a chair. If you're right-handed, you may find it easier to measure pressure in your left arm and vice versa. Be consistent with which arm you use.

2. Find your pulse by pressing firmly on the inside of your elbow,

above the bend. If you can't find it, you're pressing either too hard or too soft.

3. Wrap the cuff around your bare arm, about 2 inches (5 centimeters) above your elbow bend. The inflatable portion of the cuff should wrap all the way around your arm and fit snugly. A standard cuff works for most adults. It's designed for an arm circumference of 9 to 12 inches (23 to 30.5 centimeters). Smaller and larger cuffs also are available.

4. If you're using a stethoscope, put the flat side firmly and directly over your main artery, just below the cuff. If your monitor has a built-in stethoscope (sometimes marked with an arrow), place the stethoscope over the area where you located your pulse. Gently place the earpieces of the stethoscope into your ears.

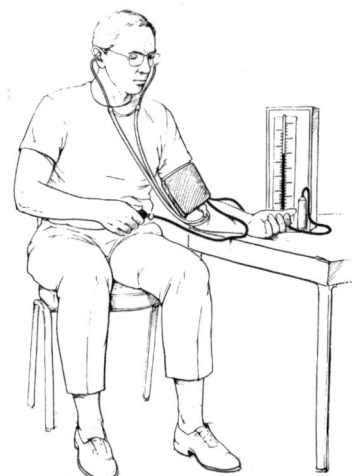

5. Put the gauge where you can easily read it, and make sure it registers at zero before you inflate the cuff.

6. Squeeze the hand bulb repeatedly to pump air into the cuff. (Use the hand of the uncuffed arm.) Inflate the cuff about 30 millimeters (mm) above your usual systolic pressure (upper number), then stop. You shouldn't hear your pulse when listening through the stethoscope.

7. Turn the release valve and slowly deflate the cuff—2 to 3 mm per second. Watch the gauge and listen carefully. When you hear the first tapping sound of your pulse, note the reading on the gauge. (The gauge's needle may jerk slightly.) This is your systolic pressure.

8. Continue deflating the cuff. When the pulse sounds stop, note the gauge's reading. This is your diastolic pressure. For some people, the pulse doesn't completely disappear, but it will fade noticeably. That sudden drop in sound marks the diastolic pressure.

9. Wait 2 minutes and repeat the procedure to check for accuracy. If you have trouble getting consistent readings, call your doctor. The problem may be your technique or equipment. Also contact your doctor if you notice an unusual or persistent increase in your blood pressure.

10. Keep a log of your blood pressure readings, along with the time and date, and show it to your doctor during your next appointment.

> **To create an electronic log, visit Mayo Clinic Health Oasis**
> Check out our Web site at *www.mayohealth.org* to see how you can easily keep track of your blood pressure measurements on your home computer. When it's time for your next appointment, simply print a copy to take with you. You'll find the blood pressure log in the Heart Center.

Using your medications wisely

If you're taking medication to control your blood pressure, remember its effectiveness depends in large part on you. When, how and with what you take your pills are important.

Taking your medication correctly

You need to take your pills as prescribed. That may sound obvious, but by some estimates only half of people taking high blood pressure medication do so in correct doses at the right time.

If you take your pills too early, you increase the level of the drug in your blood. This overdose can produce symptoms and side effects such as nausea and diarrhea, which can ruin your day. If you take your pills too late, drug levels decrease and your blood pressure may increase. And if you stop taking your pills entirely, your blood pressure may rebound to levels higher than before your condition was diagnosed.

Here are some tips to help you take your medication properly:

Tie your medication to daily events. If you have a morning medication, put the pills near your breakfast dishes, toothbrush or razor, if this doesn't endanger children or animals. Otherwise, put a sticker near these items to remind you to take your pills.

Set an alarm clock or wristwatch. The alarm will remind you when it's time to take your medication.

Use a plastic pillbox. If you take several drugs, purchase a pillbox with one to three compartments for each day of the week. Load the box once a week to help you keep track of which pills you take and when.

Ask for help from a loved one. Ask him or her to remind you to take your pills, at least until you incorporate the habit into your daily routine.

Take your pills with water. Water helps dissolve the drug. If you generally take your pills with another liquid, check with your doctor or pharmacist to make sure it mixes well with the medication. If you're supposed to take your pills with food, do so. Otherwise the drug may not be absorbed properly into your bloodstream.

Seek good lighting. Don't take your medication in the dark. You might unintentionally take the wrong pill.

Keep the original containers. Occasionally take them to your doctor to make sure you're taking the right drug in the proper dosage.

Note any side effects. Pass this information on to your doctor during your next checkup. Your doctor may want to adjust the dosage or try a different medication. All blood pressure medicine can produce side effects. However, with the right medication, most people experience few problems.

Refill your prescriptions in advance. Plan at least a couple of weeks ahead, in case the unexpected upsets your routine. Snowstorms, the flu and accidents are just a few examples of surprises that can delay your trip to the pharmacy.

Don't change your dosage. If your blood pressure increases even though you're taking your medication properly, don't increase the dosage on your own. Talk with your doctor first. Also don't decrease your dosage without first consulting your doctor.

Preventing drug interactions

There are more than 80 medications to control high blood pressure. Some can produce dangerous side effects if they're mixed with other prescription drugs, over-the-counter medicines, alternative health products, illicit drugs and even some foods. So it's important that you tell your doctor about all the medications you're taking, and to ask about any potentially harmful interactions.

Prescription drugs. Because many prescription drugs can interfere with certain blood pressure medications, tell your doctor about all of the medications you're taking. Combining two drugs that shouldn't be taken together can lead to a possibly life-threatening drug interaction.

Over-the-counter products. Pain relievers, decongestants and diet pills pose the most widespread problem if you're taking blood pressure medication. If you take some of these over-the-counter products with certain blood pressure drugs, your blood pressure may increase.

> ### Will I ever be able to stop taking medication?
> You've taken your medication faithfully and your blood pressure is within a normal range again. Now you're wondering if you'll one day be able to stop using it. The answer most likely is "no."
>
> Although some people with high blood pressure are able to reduce the amount of medication they take daily, most people continue to take medication the rest of their lives. Blood pressure drugs ensure that your blood pressure stays at a safe level and they lower your risk of stroke, heart attack and other complications of uncontrolled high blood pressure.
>
> In a few cases, people with stage 1 high blood pressure who've maintained a normal blood pressure for at least a year can discontinue their medication. To do this, your doctor needs to set up a plan for gradually reducing your medication. He or she also will want to see you frequently to make sure your blood pressure doesn't increase again.
>
> To successfully manage your blood pressure without medication, controlling your weight, staying active, eating well and limiting alcohol are essential. Some people who taper off blood pressure drugs eventually need to go back on medication.
>
> If unpleasant side effects are your main reason for wanting to discontinue your medication, a better solution is to work with your doctor to find a way to reduce or eliminate the side effects.

Anti-inflammatory drugs. Aspirin, ibuprofen (Advil, Motrin-IB), ketoprofen (Actron, Orudis-KT) and naproxen sodium (Aleve, Naprosyn) can interfere with three types of blood pressure medication: diuretics, beta blockers and angiotensin-converting enzyme (ACE) inhibitors.

Taken occasionally, anti-inflammatory drugs aren't a problem. But when used regularly, they can cause your body to retain salt and fluid, counteracting the effects of diuretics. They also can prevent the production and release of chemicals that relax your blood vessels, counteracting the effects of beta blockers. And they can reduce the ability of ACE inhibitors to widen your blood vessels.

If you take an anti-inflammatory drug for arthritis or another health problem, talk with your doctor. Your doctor may decide to change your blood pressure medication.

Cold and allergy medicine. Use these products sparingly if you have high blood pressure. They contain pseudoephedrine (a decongestant) and phenylephrine (used in nose sprays). Pseudoephedrine and phenylephrine mimic the effects of the hormone norepinephrine (noradrenaline), causing your blood vessels to narrow. This effect can increase your blood pressure.

Diet pills. They contain phenylpropanolamine, which works in the same manner as pseudoephedrine and phenylephrine.

Illicit drugs. Cocaine narrows and inflames your blood vessels and interferes with the effects of blood pressure medications. Other illegal drugs also can cause dangerous drug interactions. Part of the reason is that the manufacture of these drugs isn't regulated, and they may contain dangerous hidden substances, such as herbicides or talc.

Food. Grapefruit juice can interfere with your liver's ability to remove certain calcium antagonists from your blood. This causes the drug to build up in your body, which can lead to annoying or harmful side effects. If you take the drugs felodipine, nifedipine or verapamil, don't take them with grapefruit juice or drink grapefruit juice 2 hours before or after you take your medication.

Natural licorice, the bittersweet ingredient added to chewing tobacco and licorice cough drops, can increase your blood pressure because it contains glycyrrhizic acid. This acid makes your kidneys retain salt and fluid. If you take a diuretic to remove excess salt and fluids, avoid natural licorice. Artificially flavored licorice—the kind used in candy—isn't a problem.

Reducing medication costs

Many blood pressure medications are expensive. And taking a drug every day for the rest of your life is a costly prospect—one that's magnified if you take two or more drugs daily. However, there are ways you can reduce your medication costs.

Generic drugs. Once a pharmaceutical company's patent on a drug expires—usually after 17 years—other companies are free to make the drug from the same ingredients. This competition often spurs the original supplier to reduce the price. Plus, the cost of the new generic brands is usually lower still. The major reason is that generic manufacturers don't have to recoup costs from years of research and development.

Nutritional and herbal supplements

Alternative health products are becoming increasingly popular. But they aren't always effective or safe. This list includes products promoted to control blood pressure and those that can increase it. If you're taking a supplement—or considering it—let your doctor know.

Supplement	Our thoughts and advice
Supplements promoted to lower blood pressure	
Coenzyme Q-10	No conclusive evidence it controls blood pressure
Fish oil capsules containing omega-3 fatty acids	Capsules are high in fat and calories. May produce gastrointestinal side effects, leave fishy aftertaste. Best to eat fish
Garlic	Study results mixed. No conclusive evidence it controls blood pressure
Gingko biloba	No conclusive evidence it controls blood pressure
Green tea	No conclusive evidence it controls blood pressure
Potassium, calcium and magnesium	May interfere with other medications. Magnesium supplements may cause diarrhea. Excessive potassium can interfere with heart rhythm. Best to get minerals from food
Vitamin C	No conclusive evidence it controls blood pressure
Supplements that can increase blood pressure	
Ephedrine (Ephedra)	Claims to promote weight loss, provide herbal "high." Avoid. Can cause dangerous rise in blood pressure and heart rate
Licorice root	Claims to cure ulcers, coughs and colds. Avoid. Can increase blood pressure
Yohimbine	Claims to increase sexual desire. Avoid. Can increase blood pressure

Ask your doctor if it's OK for you to take a generic drug. And don't be surprised if the new pills look different from the original. Generic drugs are often another shape and color. Because of this, read the label carefully to make sure that the dosage for taking the medication is the same as it was for the original drug.

Generic drugs don't face the same rigorous testing as brand names. But the Food and Drug Administration does check to see if the new pills contain the same active ingredients and if they're adequately absorbed into your body. Generic drugs also must meet the same standards of identity, strength, quality and purity as required for brand name products. Still, it's a good idea to monitor your blood pressure more frequently when you first start taking a generic drug.

Splitting pills. Pills generally come in various doses. And many times higher-dose pills cost only a small amount more than lower-dose versions. This means, for example, if you need 50-milligram tablets, you can buy 100-milligram tablets, split them in half and save money.

This doesn't work, however, for capsules containing sustained-release granules. The various ingredients aren't evenly distributed on each side of the capsule. Nor should you split pills that are coated to keep them from dissolving in your stomach. Cutting them in half negates the coating's effect. In addition, the medication you take may not come in a larger dose that can be evenly divided. The pills must be cut into equal proportions.

Check with your doctor or pharmacist before splitting your pills to make sure it's safe to do so. You can purchase an inexpensive pill splitter at medical supply stores and some pharmacies. It's more convenient and accurate than using a knife and a cutting board.

Buying in bulk. In addition to comparison shopping for the best buy among pharmacies, check with discount mail-order pharmacies. Many of these are reputable firms endorsed by respected groups such as the American Association of Retired Persons.

Prices at discount suppliers are usually 10 percent to 35 percent lower than you'll find at some pharmacies. The discount is available because the clearinghouse buys and sells in bulk.

A disadvantage of buying in bulk is that if you stockpile too much medication, some of it may expire before you can use it. If your doctor changes your medication you also may end up with medication you can't use. It's best to buy enough for only 3 to 6 months. If, after receiving the medication, you discover you won't be able to use it all before the expiration date, many companies will exchange the pills.

There's another important disadvantage to buying from mail-order suppliers. You miss having a pharmacist who becomes familiar with your history and all of the medications you're taking. However, if you're diligent about keeping your doctors updated on your medications, discount suppliers can provide a safe and wallet-friendly alternative.

Combination drugs. Some blood pressure medications are used together so often that manufacturers have combined the ingredients into single tablets. These combination tablets are usually less expensive than buying the pills individually. If you take more than one blood pressure medication, ask your doctor if the medications come in combination form. A sample of combination drugs is listed in Chapter 10 (page 136).

Assistance programs. Some social service organizations and pharmaceutical companies offer free medication or drugs at greatly reduced prices to people facing financial hardship. Your doctor can help refer you to the appropriate social services group or drug manufacturer.

A list of participating pharmaceutical companies is available from the Directory of Prescription Drug Indigent Programs, published by the Pharmaceutical Manufacturers Association, and from the free brochure "Drugs, Free or Low-Cost," published by the American Heart Association.

Getting regular follow-up care

If you have stage 1 high blood pressure and no evidence of organ damage, your doctor will want to see you again within 1 to 2 months after making a diagnosis. During that first follow-up visit your doctor will evaluate your progress—determine whether your blood pressure has decreased—and ask about any side effects if you're taking medication.

If your blood pressure hasn't decreased, your doctor may make some changes in your therapy, and possibly change your medication.

If you have stage 2 or 3 high blood pressure or other medical problems that complicate your treatment, you may need to see your doctor every 2 to 4 weeks until you have your blood pressure under control.

Once your blood pressure is well controlled, a visit to your doctor once or twice a year is often all that's needed, unless you have a coexisting medical problem, such as diabetes, high cholesterol or heart or kidney disease. Then, you'll need to see your doctor more frequently.

Follow-up visits typically involve two blood pressure measurements, a general physical examination and some routine tests. The tests can alert your doctor to possible problems resulting from your medication or to a decline in your heart or kidney function related to your high blood pressure. In addition, follow-up visits are a good time to talk with your doctor about issues related to your weight, diet or activity level.

Unfortunately, close to half of people with high blood pressure don't see their doctor regularly as recommended. This may be another reason why most Americans with high blood pressure aren't in control of their condition.

Reaching your goal

If you're having trouble lowering your blood pressure to a safe level, you may be tempted to give up. But don't. For some people, reaching a normal or optimal blood pressure level simply takes time.

You can help by:
- Learning all you can about high blood pressure. Because you're reading this book, you're already well on your way.
- Practicing good lifestyle habits, such as controlling your weight, eating healthfully, being physically active and limiting alcohol
- Remaining patient and optimistic

Your family and friends

Educating your family and friends about high blood pressure is also important to helping you manage your condition. If they don't understand the danger that uncontrolled high blood pressure poses to your health, they may unintentionally work against you. This might include offering you unhealthful food, pestering you about the time you spend on physical activities and even complaining about the high cost of your medicine.

If your family and friends fully understand that your life is at risk if you don't control your blood pressure, they can help make sure you eat well and remind you when it's time to take your medication or to go for your daily walk. In fact, they may even join you.

Your family and friends can become your most loyal allies in helping you control your blood pressure. That's why it's important that you ask for and welcome their support.

A lifelong endeavor

There is no cure for high blood pressure. You'll always have it. But you can make a big difference in how the disease affects your life. Much of the responsibility for controlling your high blood pressure is yours. Through changes in your lifestyle and, if necessary, medication, you can take charge of your blood pressure and avoid or reduce the disease's dangerous effects.

Your future health depends on you.

Wrap-up

Key points to remember from this chapter:
- Monitoring your blood pressure at home can help you stay in control of your condition. You can purchase blood pressure monitors at medical supply stores and some pharmacies.
- If you take blood pressure medication, it's essential that you take it as directed every day. Pillboxes and daily reminders can help you take your pills correctly.
- Generic drugs, buying in bulk, splitting your pills or purchasing combination drugs may be possible options for reducing your medication costs. Assistance programs also are available if your financial resources are limited.
- Over-the-counter pain relievers, sinus and allergy drugs and diet pills can interfere with some blood pressure medications.
- See your doctor regularly as recommended.
- Enlist the support of your family and friends to help you stay in control.
- Controlling high blood pressure is a lifelong pursuit.

Menus With DASH

The pages that follow include a week of menus developed by Mayo Clinic dietitians, based on the recommendations of the Dietary Approaches to Stop Hypertension (DASH) eating plan.

The menus emphasize grains, vegetables, fruits and low-fat dairy products. This variety helps provide plentiful amounts of the minerals potassium, calcium and magnesium, which are associated with lower blood pressure, plus fiber. Each day's menu is based on a diet of 2,000 calories, with no more than 30 percent of calories coming from fat. (See page 61 to determine your calorie needs. A registered dietitian can help you adjust the menus to meet your calorie level.) In addition, sodium is limited to 2,400 milligrams a day.

Accompanying each of the menus is the recipe for the dinner entrée. The recipes use commonly available ingredients and are designed with an eye toward ease of preparation.

Use these menus as a guide to adopting a more nutritiously balanced diet. Feel free to make substitutions or adjustments to the menus to suit your tastes. If, for example, you don't care for peaches, you can substitute the peach in Day 1's menu with another fruit, such as an apple or serving of strawberries.

The idea is to learn to enjoy a variety of foods in your daily diet.

Day 1

Breakfast
2 oatmeal pancakes, topped with ½ cup (4 oz./125 g) unsweetened applesauce
1 cup (8 oz./250 g) low-fat fruit-flavored yogurt
Decaffeinated coffee

Lunch
BBQ beef sandwich: 2 ounces (60 g) thin-sliced roast beef, topped with 1 tablespoon BBQ sauce, on a toasted onion roll
1 small ear of corn or ½ cup (3 oz./90 g) corn kernels
Mixed greens
2 tablespoons light cucumber dressing
1 fresh peach
1 cup (8 fl. oz./250 mL) fat-free milk

Dinner
Honey Chicken on Apricot Wild Rice (see recipe, page 175)
Steamed asparagus (4 to 6 spears)
1 country-style biscuit
1 teaspoon soft margarine
½ tomato, sliced with fresh cilantro
½ cup (2 oz./60 g) mixed fresh berries
Hot herbal tea

Snack (anytime)
1 muffin
¾ cup (6 fl. oz./180 mL) orange juice

Food servings — *Grains* 8; *Fruits* 4; *Vegetables* 5; *Dairy products* 2; *Poultry, seafood, meat* 2; *Legumes/nuts* 0; *Fats* 2; *Sweets* 0

Nutritional analysis — *Calories* 2,039 (*Kilojoules* 8,564); *Fat* 40 g; *Saturated fat* 16 g; *Cholesterol* 170 mg; *Sodium* 2,183 mg; *Fiber* 31 g

---

Menu-planning tip
By removing the skin from the chicken as called for in the recipe for Honey Chicken on Apricot Wild Rice, you save 50 calories and about 5 grams of fat.

Day 2

Breakfast
1 cup (1½ oz./45 g) bran cereal, topped with ½ cup (3 oz./90 g) dried mixed fruit (apples, apricots, raisins)
2 slices whole-grain toast
1 teaspoon soft margarine
1 cup (8 fl. oz./250 mL) fat-free milk

Lunch
Turkey sandwich ala Mediterranean: ¼ cup (1 oz./30 g) cooked turkey, topped with 1 ounce (30 g) part-skim mozzarella cheese, ½ sliced tomato and 2 tablespoons commercially available pesto sauce, on 2 slices whole-wheat bread
1 kiwifruit
Mixed greens tossed with vinegar and 1 teaspoon olive oil
¾ cup (6 fl. oz./180 mL) unsalted vegetable juice

Dinner
Poached Salmon With Melon Salsa (see recipe, page 176)
Roasted red-skinned potatoes (3 small)
1 whole-wheat roll
1 tablespoon honey
1 cup (8 fl. oz./250 mL) fat-free milk

Snack (anytime)
1 apple
⅓ cup (1 oz./30 g) unsalted nuts
¼ cup (½ oz./15 g) unsalted pretzels

Food servings — *Grains 8; Fruits 4; Vegetables 4; Dairy products 3; Poultry, seafood, meat 1½; Legumes/nuts 1; Fats 3; Sweets 1*

Nutritional analysis — *Calories 2,010 (Kilojoules 8,442); Fat 62 g; Saturated fat 12 g; Cholesterol 112 mg; Sodium 1,725 mg; Fiber 30 g*

Menu-planning tip
One kiwifruit provides 74 milligrams of vitamin C, all of your day's recommendations for vitamin C.

Day 3

Breakfast
1 cup (6 oz./185 g) mixed fruits (melons, banana, apple, berries), topped with 1 cup (8 oz./250 g) low-fat vanilla-flavored yogurt and ⅓ cup (1 oz./30 g) toasted almonds
1 bran muffin
1 cup (8 fl. oz./250 mL) fat-free milk
Herbal tea

Lunch
Curried chicken wrap: 1 medium flour tortilla filled with mixture of ⅓ cup (2 oz./60 g) cooked chopped chicken, ½ chopped apple, 2 tablespoons fat-free mayonnaise and ½ teaspoon curry powder
1 cup (4 oz./125 g) raw baby carrots
2 reduced-sodium rye crackers
1 nectarine
1 cup (8 fl. oz./250 mL) fat-free milk

Dinner
Basil and Sun-Dried Tomato Fettuccine (see recipe, page 177)
Mixed greens
2 tablespoons low-fat Caesar dressing
1 whole-wheat roll
1 teaspoon margarine
Sparkling water

Snack (anytime)
Trail mix made with 2 tablespoons raisins, ¾ cup (1½ oz./45 g) unsalted mini-pretzels and ⅓ cup (1 oz./30 g) unsalted nuts

Food servings — *Grains* 7; *Fruits* 5; *Vegetables* 4; *Dairy products* 3; *Poultry, seafood, meat* 1; *Legumes/nuts* 2; *Fats* 2; *Sweets* 1

Nutritional analysis — *Calories* 2,109 (*Kilojoules* 8,858); *Fat* 59 g; *Saturated fat* 8 g; *Cholesterol* 61 mg; *Sodium* 1,310 mg; *Fiber* 30 g

---

Menu-planning tip
Eating more meals that don't include meat, such as this evening's Basil and Sun-Dried Tomato Fettuccine, can help lower both your blood pressure and your blood cholesterol. People who follow plant-based diets tend to have a lower risk for high blood pressure and heart disease.

Day 4

Breakfast
1 whole-wheat bagel
2 tablespoons peanut butter
1 medium orange
1 cup (8 fl. oz./250 mL) fat-free milk
Decaffeinated coffee

Lunch
Spinach salad: fresh spinach leaves mixed with 1 sliced pear, ½ cup
 (3 oz./90 g) mandarin orange sections, ⅓ cup (1 oz./30 g) unsalted
 peanuts and 2 tablespoons fat-free red wine vinaigrette
12 reduced-sodium wheat crackers
1 cup (8 fl. oz./250 mL) fat-free milk

Dinner
Sweet Potato and Shrimp Gumbo (see recipe, page 178)
1 sourdough roll
1 teaspoon soft margarine
1 cup (4 oz./125 g) fresh berries with chopped mint
Herbal iced tea

Snack (anytime)
1 cup (8 oz./250 g) fat-free yogurt
8 vanilla wafers

Food servings — *Grains 7; Fruits 5; Vegetables 4; Dairy products 3; Poultry, seafood, meat 1; Legumes/nuts 2; Fats 1; Sweets 0*

Nutritional analysis — *Calories 1,997 (Kilojoules 8,387); Fat 55 g; Saturated fat 7 g; Cholesterol 78 mg; Sodium 1,523 mg; Fiber 32 g*

Menu-planning tip
Adding a pear and mandarin oranges to your spinach salad is an easy way to include more fruit in your diet. When combined with a glass of orange juice for breakfast, you've already tallied three fruit servings by lunch. These fruits also contain moderate to high amounts of potassium.

Day 5

Breakfast
1 cup (6 oz./185 g) cooked old-fashioned oatmeal, topped with 1 tablespoon brown sugar
2 slices whole-wheat toast
1 teaspoon soft margarine
1 banana
1 cup (8 fl. oz./250 mL) fat-free milk

Lunch
Tuna salad: ½ cup (5 oz./155 g) drained, unsalted water-packed tuna, mixed with 2 tablespoons fat-free mayonnaise, 15 grapes and ¼ cup (1 oz./30 g) diced celery, served on Romaine lettuce
12 low-sodium wheat crackers
1 cup (8 fl. oz./250 mL) fat-free milk

Dinner
Teriyaki Vegetable and Beef Kabobs (see recipe, page 179)
1 cup (6 oz./180 g) steamed rice with parsley
⅛ (or 2 rings) pineapple
Green tea

Snack (anytime)
1 cup (8 oz./250 g) low-fat yogurt
1 banana

Food servings — *Grains* 8; *Fruits* 4; *Vegetables* 4; *Dairy products* 3; *Poultry, seafood, meat* 2; *Legumes/nuts* 0; *Fats* 2; *Sweets* 1

Nutritional analysis — *Calories* 2,010 (*Kilojoules* 8,442); *Fat* 40 g; *Saturated fat* 6 g; *Cholesterol* 190 mg; *Sodium* 1,950 mg; *Fiber* 33 g

---

Menu-planning tip
A simple way to ensure 3 servings of dairy foods is to include an 8-ounce glass of fat-free milk with each meal. Or, as in today's menu, substitute low-fat yogurt for an equal amount of calcium. Dairy products are rich in calcium—a mineral that can help control blood pressure and help keep your bones and teeth strong.

Day 6

Breakfast
1 English muffin
2 tablespoons fat-free cream cheese
1 cup (4 oz./125 g) fresh strawberries
1 cup (8 fl. oz./250 mL) fat-free milk

Lunch
Lemon peppered chicken breast on rye: ½ grilled boneless chicken breast seasoned with lemon pepper, topped with shredded lettuce and 1 tablespoon low-fat mayonnaise, on 2 slices rye bread
1 cup (4 oz./125 g) fresh vegetables (raw baby carrots, celery sticks, broccoli florets)
2 reduced-sodium rye crackers
¾ cup (6 fl. oz./180 mL) cranberry juice

Dinner
Rosemary Lamb and White Beans (see recipe, page 180)
1 cup (6 oz./180 g) steamed broccoli florets
1 slice whole-wheat bread
1 teaspoon soft margarine
1 fresh sliced pear sprinkled with balsamic vinegar
1 cup (8 fl. oz./250 mL) fat-free milk

Snack (anytime)
1 cup (8 oz./250 g) low-fat cottage cheese
2 fresh apricots
4 graham crackers

Food servings — *Grains 8; Fruits 4; Vegetables 4; Dairy products 3; Poultry, seafood, meat 2; Legumes/nuts 2; Fats 3; Sweets 0*

Nutritional analysis — *Calories 1,902 (Kilojoules 7,988); Fat 35 g; Saturated fat 4 g; Cholesterol 165 mg; Sodium 2,365 mg; Fiber 33 g*

Menu-planning tip
The DASH diet recommends 4 to 5 servings of legumes, nuts or seeds each week. The white beans in this evening's meal provide 2 servings of legumes—half of your weekly goal. Beans are low in fat and cholesterol-free. They also supply plentiful amounts of fiber, protein, potassium, calcium and magnesium.

Day 7

Breakfast
Southwestern omelet: 1 egg + 2 egg whites, 1½ ounces (45 g) low-fat cheddar cheese, ¼ cup (1 oz./30 g) chopped green or red bell peppers, ¼ cup (1½ oz./45 g) chopped tomato
1 medium cornmeal muffin
2 teaspoons fruit spread
¾ cup (6 fl. oz./180 mL) orange juice
Decaffeinated coffee

Lunch
Vegetable pita: 1 whole-wheat pita stuffed with shredded lettuce, ½ chopped tomato, ¼ sliced cucumber, ⅓ cup (1½ oz./45 g) feta cheese and 2 tablespoons light French dressing
10 cherries
1 cup (8 oz./250 g) frozen yogurt
Herbal tea

Dinner
Cruciferous Stir-Fry Over Rice (see recipe, page 181)
1 slice crusty bread
1 teaspoon soft margarine
1 fresh peach sprinkled with cinnamon
1 cup (8 fl. oz./250 mL) fat-free milk

Snack (anytime)
2 cups (1 oz./30 g) unsalted air-popped popcorn
¾ cup (6 fl. oz./180 mL) cranberry juice

Food servings — *Grains* 8; *Fruits* 4; *Vegetables* 5; *Dairy products* 3; *Poultry, seafood, meat* 1; *Legumes/nuts* 1; *Fats* 3; *Sweets* 1

Nutritional analysis — *Calories* 1,957 (*Kilojoules* 8,219); *Fat* 52 g; *Saturated fat* 19 g; *Cholesterol* 297 mg; *Sodium* 2,209 mg; *Fiber* 25 g

---

Menu-planning tip
This evening's Cruciferous Stir-Fry Over Rice includes seasonings from the Orient. Orange zest, five-spice powder, ginger, garlic and zesty red pepper flakes eliminate the need for salty soy sauce.

Honey Chicken on Apricot Wild Rice

Honey Chicken
Serves: 6 — Preparation: 10 minutes — Cooking: 40 minutes

3 tablespoons wheat germ
2 tablespoons honey
1 tablespoon Dijon mustard
1 tablespoon canned apricot nectar or apricot jam
¾ teaspoon reduced-sodium soy sauce
6 skinless, bone-in chicken breast halves, 5 oz. (155 g) each, trimmed of visible fat

Preheat an oven to 375 F (190 C).

In a small bowl, mix together the wheat germ, honey, mustard, apricot nectar or jam and soy sauce until well blended.

Arrange the chicken pieces, bone side down, on a baking sheet. Spread the wheat germ mixture evenly over the chicken breasts. Bake until the chicken is opaque throughout and the wheat germ mixture has formed a crust, 35-40 minutes.

To serve, divide the rice among individual plates. Top each with a chicken breast half.

Per Serving — *Calories* 411 (*Kilojoules* 1,721); *Protein* 36 g; *Carbohydrates* 63 g; *Fat* 2 g; *Saturated Fat* <1 g; *Cholesterol* 63 mg; *Sodium* 163 mg; *Fiber* 5 g

Apricot Wild Rice
Makes: 6 cups (2 lb/1 kg) — Preparation: 20 minutes — Cooking: 1 hour

1 oz. (30 g) dried shiitake mushrooms, stemmed
1½ cups (12 fl. oz./375 mL) warm water
2 cups (12 oz./375 g) wild rice, rinsed in a fine-mesh sieve under cold running water
½ cup (3 oz./90 g) coarsely chopped dried apricots
2 shallots, minced

In a small bowl, soak the mushrooms in the warm water until barely softened, about 20 minutes. Remove the mushrooms, reserving the liquid. Coarsely chop the mushrooms. Strain the mushroom-soaking liquid through a fine-mesh sieve into a measuring cup. Add enough water to equal 5 cups (40 fl. oz./1.25 L) liquid. Pour the liquid into a large saucepan and bring to a boil. Add the wild rice, mushrooms, apricots, and shallots. Return to a boil, cover and reduce heat to low. Cool until the rice is tender and all the liquid has been absorbed, 45 minutes to 1 hour.

Per Serving — *Calories* 252 (*Kilojoules* 1,056); *Protein* 9 g; *Carbohydrates* 55 g; *Fat* <1 g; *Saturated Fat* <1 g; *Cholesterol* 0 mg; *Sodium* 6 mg; *Fiber* 5 g

Poached Salmon With Melon Salsa

Poached Salmon
Serves: 6 — Preparation: 40 minutes — Cooking: 15 minutes

2 green (spring) onions, thinly sliced, including green portions
1½ teaspoons chopped fresh mint
1 teaspoon grated fresh ginger
3 tablespoons grated lime zest
1½ lb. (750 g) salmon fillets, skinned and cut into 6 pieces

Preheat an oven to 450 F (230 C).

In a small bowl, toss together the onions, mint, ginger and lime zest.

Place 6 pieces of aluminum foil, each 10 inches (25 cm) square, onto a work surface. Place a piece of salmon in the center of each square. Top each with an equal amount of the onion mixture. Fold in the edges of the foil and crimp to seal. Place the packets in a single layer on a baking sheet and bake until opaque throughout, 12-15 minutes.

Melon Salsa
1 honeydew melon, about 3 lb. (1.5 kg), peeled, seeded, and cut into ½-inch (12-mm) cubes
1 yellow bell pepper (capsicum), seeded, stemmed and cut into ½-inch (12-mm) squares
¼ cup (2 fl. oz./60 mL) lime juice
½ red (Spanish) onion, chopped
1 jalapeño chile, minced
2 tablespoons chopped fresh mint

To make the salsa, in a medium bowl, toss together the melon, pepper, lime juice, onion, jalapeño and mint.

To serve, transfer the contents of each packet onto an individual plate. Top each with an equal amount of the salsa.

Per Serving — *Calories* 261 (*Kilojoules* 1,093); *Protein* 24 g; *Carbohydrates* 14 g; *Fat* 12 g; *Saturated Fat* 2 g; *Cholesterol* 67 mg; *Sodium* 83 mg; *Fiber* 2 g

Basil and Sun-Dried Tomato Fettuccine

Serves: 6 — Preparation: 15 minutes — Cooking: 15 minutes

⅓ cup (3 fl. oz./80 mL) canned vegetable broth
⅓ cup (3 fl. oz./80 mL) water
6 sun-dried tomatoes (not oil-packed), cut into thin strips
2 teaspoons olive oil
2 garlic cloves, crushed with a garlic press
¼ teaspoon red pepper flakes
12 oz. (375 g) dried fettuccine or linguine
½ cup (¾ oz./20 g) lightly packed torn basil leaves
2 tablespoons grated Parmesan cheese
1 tablespoon dried bread crumbs

In a small saucepan over medium heat, bring the vegetable broth, water, sun-dried tomatoes, olive oil, garlic and red pepper flakes to a boil. Remove from heat, cover and keep warm.

Fill a large pot three-quarters full of water and bring to a boil. Add the pasta and cook until al dente, about 10 minutes, or according to package directions. Remove ¼ cup (2 fl. oz./60 mL) of the cooking water, then drain the pasta thoroughly.

In a warmed serving bowl, combine the pasta, broth mixture, basil and reserved cooking water. Toss to combine, and coat the pasta evenly with the sauce.

To make dried bread crumbs, choose a loaf of whole-wheat bread with a firm, course-textured crumb. If you want a finer consistency to the crumbs, trim away the crusts. With your hands, crumble the bread into a blender or food processor. Pulse the machine on and off until the crumbs reach the desired consistency. If you like drier crumbs for a crunchier consistency, spread them in a baking dish or on a baking sheet and put them in an oven set at its lowest temperature. Bake for about 1 hour, stirring occasionally, or until they feel thoroughly dry to the touch.

To serve, divide among individual plates. Top each with an equal amount of the Parmesan and bread crumbs.

Per Serving — *Calories* 247 (*Kilojoules* 1,033); *Protein* 9 g; *Carbohydrates* 45 g; *Fat* 3 g; *Saturated Fat* <1 g; *Cholesterol* 1 mg; *Sodium* 103 mg; *Fiber* 2 g

Sweet Potato and Shrimp Gumbo

Serves: 6 — Preparation: 25 minutes — Cooking: 30 minutes

¾ cup (6 fl. oz./180 mL) tomato juice
1 onion, chopped
1 green bell pepper (capsicum), stemmed, seeded and chopped
½ lb. (250 g) okra, stemmed and thinly sliced
2 celery stalks, chopped
⅔ cup (5 fl. oz./160 mL) dry white wine
¼ cup (2 fl. oz./60 mL) distilled white vinegar
1 lb. (500 g) sweet potatoes, peeled and cut into 1-inch (2.5-cm) cubes
3 cups (28 oz./875 g) canned crushed tomatoes or tomato purée
1½ tablespoons chili powder
⅛ teaspoon cayenne pepper
24 fresh or thawed frozen shrimp (prawns), shelled and deveined
6 cups (32 oz./1 kg) cooked, hot white rice

In a large frying pan over medium-high heat, heat the tomato juice. Add the onion, bell pepper, okra and celery and sauté until wilted and softened slightly, 5-7 minutes.

Add the wine and vinegar and bring to a boil. Stir in the sweet potatoes, tomatoes or purée, chili powder and cayenne and cook until it returns to a boil. Reduce heat to low, cover and simmer, stirring occasionally, until the sweet potatoes are tender, 15-18 minutes.

Add the shrimp and stir to combine. Cover and cook until the shrimp are pink, about 5 minutes.

To serve, divide the rice among individual bowls. Top each with an equal amount of the gumbo.

Per Serving — *Calories* 362 (*Kilojoules* 1,516); *Protein* 14 g; *Carbohydrates* 72 g; *Fat* 2 g; *Saturated Fat* <1 g; *Cholesterol* 49 mg; *Sodium* 397 mg; *Fiber* 6 g

Teriyaki Vegetable and Beef Kabobs

Serves: 6 — Preparation: 25 minutes — Marinating: 30 minutes — Cooking: 10 minutes

Marinade
½ cup (4 fl. oz./125 mL) reduced-sodium soy sauce
4 garlic cloves, crushed with a garlic press
2 teaspoons grated fresh ginger
2 teaspoons lime juice
2 teaspoons honey
¼ teaspoon red pepper flakes
¼ teaspoon sesame oil

1 lb. (500 g) beef tenderloin, trimmed of visible fat and cut into 1-inch (2.5-cm) cubes
3 Japanese eggplants (aubergines), cut crosswise into ½-inch (12-mm) pieces
1¼ lb. (625 g) white mushrooms
2 zucchini (courgettes), cut crosswise into ½-inch (12-mm) pieces
2 yellow squash, cut crosswise into ½-inch (12-mm) pieces
2 red bell peppers (capsicums), stemmed, seeded and cut into ¾-inch (2-cm) squares
2 red (Spanish) onions, cut into ½-inch-thick (12-mm) wedges

To make the marinade, in a large bowl, whisk together the soy sauce, garlic, ginger, lime juice, honey, pepper flakes and sesame oil. Transfer 3 tablespoons of the marinade to a medium bowl. Add the beef to the medium bowl, tossing to coat. Add the eggplants, mushrooms, zucchini, squash, peppers and onions to the large bowl, tossing to coat.

Cover and marinate both the meat and vegetables at room temperature for 30 minutes, tossing once or twice.

Meanwhile, preheat a broiler (griller). Line the broiler pan with aluminum foil and coat with nonstick cooking spray. Soak 18 long wooden skewers in water to cover.

Using a slotted spoon, remove the meat and vegetables from the bowls and pat dry with paper towels. Discard the meat marinade.

For the 6 beef kabobs, divide the meat cubes equally among 6 skewers, threading it alternately with one third of the mushrooms, zucchini, squash, peppers and onions.

For the 12 vegetable kabobs, thread the eggplant pieces onto 12 skewers, alternating with the remaining mushrooms, zucchini, squash, peppers and onions.

Working in batches if necessary, place the kabobs 2 inches (5 cm) apart on the broiler pan. Position the pan 4 inches (10 cm) from the heat source. Broil, turning once or twice and brushing the kabobs with any remaining vegetable marinade, until the vegetables are tender and the beef is nicely browned, 8-10 minutes.

To serve, place 1 beef and 2 vegetable kabobs on each plate.

Per Vegetable Kabob — *Calories* 35 (*Kilojoules* 147); *Protein* 2 g; *Carbohydrates* 7 g; *Fat* <1 g; *Saturated Fat* 0 g; *Cholesterol* 0 mg; *Sodium* 181 mg; *Fiber* 1 g

Per Beef Kabob — *Calories* 160 (*Kilojoules* 670); *Protein* 18 g; *Carbohydrates* 8 g; *Fat* 6 g; *Saturated Fat* 2 g; *Cholesterol* 48 mg; *Sodium* 393 mg; *Fiber* 1 g

Rosemary Lamb and White Beans

Serves: 6 — Preparation: 10 minutes — Marinating: 30 minutes — Cooking: 30 minutes

Rosemary Lamb
- 1½ teaspoons finely chopped fresh rosemary or ½ teaspoon dried rosemary
- 2 garlic cloves, crushed with a garlic press
- ½ teaspoon olive oil
- 6 loin lamb chops, 5 oz. (155 g) each, trimmed of visible fat

Beans
- 4½ cups (2 lb./1 kg) cooked white beans or canned white beans, rinsed and drained
- 1½ cups (9 oz./280 g) diced fresh tomatoes or canned diced tomatoes, drained
- 1 small onion, finely chopped
- ½ cup (¾ oz./20 g) chopped fresh flat-leaf (Italian) parsley
- 1½ teaspoons chopped fresh rosemary or ½ teaspoon dried rosemary
- 3 garlic cloves, minced
- ¾ teaspoon ground pepper
- 6 small rosemary sprigs

In a small bowl, combine the rosemary, garlic and olive oil. Rub the mixture evenly into both sides of the lamb chops. Cover and marinate at room temperature for 30 minutes.

For the beans, preheat an oven to 425 F (220 C). Coat a 2-qt (2-L) shallow baking dish with nonstick cooking spray.

In a large bowl, combine the beans, tomatoes, onion, parsley, rosemary, garlic and pepper.

Spread the bean mixture into the prepared dish. Cover and bake until heated through, about 15 minutes.

Meanwhile, preheat a broiler (griller). Arrange the lamb chops on a broiler pan and place the pan 4 inches (10 cm) from the heat. Broil, turning once, until lightly browned on both sides, 6-7 minutes total.

Remove the dish from the oven and arrange the lamb chops on top of the beans, pressing down gently. Return to the oven and cook, uncovered, until the beans are lightly browned on top and the chops are fully cooked, about 10 minutes.

To serve, divide the beans and lamb chops among individual plates. Garnish with the rosemary sprigs.

Per Serving — *Calories* 354 (*Kilojoules* 1,482); *Protein* 32 g; *Carbohydrates* 43 g; *Fat* 7 g; *Saturated Fat* 2 g; *Cholesterol* 51 mg; *Sodium* 61 mg; *Fiber* 7 g

Cruciferous Stir-Fry Over Rice

Serves: 6 — **Preparation: 20 minutes** — **Cooking: 20 minutes**

3½ cups (28 fl. oz./875 mL) water
1 cup (8 fl. oz./250 mL) canned vegetable broth
2 tablespoons grated orange zest
1½ teaspoons five-spice powder
3 cups (21 oz./655 g) basmati or Texmati rice
1 tablespoon canola oil
1 tablespoon minced fresh ginger
3 garlic cloves, minced
4 green (spring) onions, finely chopped, including green portions
¼ teaspoon red pepper flakes
1 lb. (500 g) broccoli, cut into florets
1 lb. (500 g) cauliflower, cut into florets
8 oz. (250 g) firm tofu, drained, blotted dry and cut into ½-inch (12-mm) cubes
8 oz. (250 g) oyster mushrooms, halved
1 tablespoon sesame seeds
1 tablespoon reduced-sodium soy sauce

In a large, heavy saucepan, bring the water, broth, orange zest and five-spice powder to a boil. Stir in the rice. When the liquid returns to a boil, cover and reduce heat to low. Simmer until the rice is tender and the liquid has been absorbed, about 18 minutes.

Remove the pan from heat and let stand 5 minutes, covered, then fluff the rice with a fork.

Meanwhile, in a wok or large nonstick frying pan over high heat, heat half the oil. Add half each of the ginger, garlic, green onions and pepper flakes, and stir-fry until fragrant, about 30 seconds. Add half the broccoli and cauliflower and stir-fry until the broccoli turns bright green, about 2 minutes.

Add half the tofu, mushrooms, sesame seeds and soy sauce, and stir-fry until the tofu is heated through and the vegetables are tender-crisp, 2-3 minutes. Transfer the mixture to a large bowl and keep warm. Repeat with the remaining ingredients.

To serve, divide the rice among individual plates. Top each with an equal amount of the vegetables and tofu.

Per Serving — *Calories* 480 *(Kilojoules* 2,007*); Protein* 22 g; *Carbohydrates* 91 g; *Fat* 9 g; *Saturated Fat* <1 g; *Cholesterol* 0 mg; *Sodium* 352 mg; *Fiber* 6 g

The recipes on pages 175-181 are used with permission from *The Mayo Clinic | Williams-Sonoma Cookbook*. Weldon Owen Inc., 1998.

High Blood Pressure Medications Guide*

Generic names	Brand names in USA	Brand names in India
Diuretics		
Thiazides		
bendroflumethiazide	Naturetin	Aprinox
chlorothiazide	Diuril	Cloride
chlorthalidone	Hygroton, Thalitone	Hythalton
hydrochlorothiazide	Esidrix, Hydrodiuril, Microzide, Oretic	Esidrex
indapamide	Lozol	Indap, Lorvas, Natrilix
methyclothiazide	Aquatensen, Enduron	Enduron
metolazone	Diulo, Mykrox, Zaroxolyn	Metenix-5
Loop		
bumetanide	Bumex	Bumet
ethacrynic acid	Edecrin	Edecrin
furosemide	Lasix	Lasix, Salinex
torsemide	Demadex	—
Potassium - Sparing		
amiloride	Midamor	Amimide, Frumil
spironolactone	Aldactone	Aldactone, Fruselac, Spiromide
triamterene	Dyrenium	Ditide, Frusemene
Beta Blockers		
acebutolol	Sectral	Sectral
atenolol	Tenormin	Altol, Catenol, Hyperten, Odinol, Presolar, Tensimin
betaxolol	Kerlone	Iobet, Nopres
bisoprolol	Zebeta	Concor
carteolol	Cartrol	—
carvedilol	Coreg	Carca, Carvidac
labetalol	Normodyne, Trandate	L-Beta, Normadate
metoprolol	Lopressor, Toprol XL	Betaloc, Metocard, Metolar, Metoprolol
nadolol	Corgard	Corgard
penbutolol	Levatol	—
pindolol	Visken	Visken
propranolol	Inderal, Inderal LA	Betabloc, Betalong, Betaspan, Cardiolong, Ciplar, Corbeta, Inderal
timolol	Blocadren	Iotim, Ocobar, Ocupres
ACE Inhibitors		
benazepril	Lotensin	Benace

*This guide has been prepared under the supervision of Dr. J. S. Bapna, Ph.D., FAMS, Director, Institute of Human Behaviour & Allied Sciences, Delhi, and a former President of the Indian Pharmacology Society.

captopril	Capoten	Aceten, Angiopril, Capotril, Inhibace
enalapril	Vasotec	ENA, Enace, Enam, Envas
fosinopril	Monopril	—
lisinopril	Prinivil, Zestril	Cipril, Linvas, Lipril, Lislo, Listril
moexipril	Univasc	—
quinapril	Accupril	—
ramipril	Altace	Cardace, Corpril, Ramace
trandolopril	Mavik	—

Angiotensin II Receptor Blockers

irbesartan	Avapro	—
losartan potassium	Cozaar	Alsartan, Angizaar, Repace, Zaart
valsartan	Diovan	—

Calcium Antagonists

amlodipine	Norvasc	Amcard, Amlopin, Amlopres, Amtas, Calchek
diltiazem	Cardizem CD, Cardizem SR, Dilacor XR, Tiazac	Altiazem, Dicard, Dilcardia, Dilzem, DTM
felodipine	Plendil	Felogard, Plendil, Renedil
isradipine	DynaCirc, DynaCirc CR	—
nicardipine	Cardene SR	—
nifedipine	Adalat CC, Procardia XL	Calcigard, Cardilat, Depin, Nifelat
verapamil	Calan SR, Covera HS, Isoptin SR, Verelan	Calaptin, Vasopten, Veramil, Verap

Alpha Blockers

doxazosin	Cardura	Duracard
prazosin	Minipress	Minipress XL GITS, Prazopress
terazosin	Hytrin	Hytrin, Olyster, Terapress

Central-Acting Agents

clonidine	Catapres	Catapres, Clothaltion
guanabenz	Wytensin	Rexitene
guanadrel	Hylorel	Hylorel
guanethidine	Ismelin	Ismelin
guanfacine	Tenex	Estulic
methyldopa	Aldomet	Aldomet, Alphadopa, Emdopa
reserpine	Serpasil	Reserpine, Serpasil

Direct Vasodilators

hydralazine	Apresoline	Hydralazine, Nepresol
minoxidil	Loniten	Gromane, Hairex, Minoxidil, Mintop

Combinations of a Diuretic & a Beta Blocker

bendroflumethiazide & nadolol	Corzide	—
chlorthalidone & atenolol	Tenoretic	Atecard-D, Tenoric-25
hydrochlorothiazide & bisoprolol	Ziac	—
hydrochlorothiazide & propranolol	Inderide LA	Betanol-D, Ciplar-H
hydrochlorothiazide & metoprolol	Lopressor HCT	Selopres

Combinations of a Diuretic & an ACE Inhibitor

hydrochlorothiazide & benazepril	Lotensin HCT	—
hydrochlorothiazide & captopril	Capozide	Acezide, Angiopril D.U., Capotril-H
hydrochlorothiazide & enalapril	Vaseretic	Enace-D, Invozide
hydrochlorothiazide & lisinopril	Prinzide, Zestoretic	Cipril-H

Combinations of a Diuretic & an Angiotensin II Receptor Antagonist

hydrochlorothiazide & losartan potassium	Hyzaar	Angizaar-H, Losar-H
hydrochlorothiazide & valsartan	Diovan HCT	—

Combinations of two Diuretics

amiloride & hydrochlorothiazide	Moduretic	Biduret, Biduret-L
spironolactone & hydrochlorothiazide	Aldactazide	Aldactide
triamterene & hydrochlorothiazide	Dyazide, Maxzide	—

Combinations of a Calcium Antagonist & an ACE Inhibitor

amlodipine & benazepril	Lotrel	—
diltiazem & enalapril	Teczem	—
verapamil & trandolopril	Tarka	—
felodipine & enalapril	Lexxel	—

Anti-inflammatory Drugs which interfere with Blood Pressure Medication

aspirin		Lodosprin, Mazoral
ibuprofen	Advil, Motrin-IB	Brufen, Ibucon, Ibugesic, Ibugin
ketoprofen	Actron, Orudis-KT	Ketofen, Ostofen, Redvfen, Rhofenid
naproxen sodium	Aleve, Naprosyn	Artagen, Nalyxan, Ralnep

Index

A

ACE inhibitors, 129–130
   and alcohol, 114
   and anti-inflammatory drugs, 160
   and coronary artery disease, 147
   and diabetes, 148
   and heart failure, 147
   and high cholesterol, 148
   and kidney disease, 130, 149
   and pregnancy, 141
Acebutolol, 128
Activity, 63–76
   aerobic, 65–67
   avoiding injury, 75–76
   duration of, 67–69
   effect on blood pressure, 63–64
   fitness plan, 69–75
   intensity of, 64–65
   motivation, 69–70, 74–75
   and stress, 120
Additives, 95
Adrenal disease, 33
Adrenaline, 14, 113, 118, 119
Aerobic activity, 65–67, 72
Age risk factor, 28–29, 57, 145
Alcohol use, 31, 90, 112–114
Allergy medicines, 161
Alpha blockers, 132–133, 135, 148
Ambulatory monitor, 42
Amiloride, 127, 136
Amlodipine, 132, 136
Anemia, 44
Aneurysm, 23, 43, 45
Angiography, 45
Angiotensin I, 129
Angiotensin II, 128, 129, 137
Angiotensin II receptor blockers,
      130–131, 141, 148
Anti-inflammatory drugs, 160
Antihypertensives, 125
Arrhythmia, 146

Arteries
   and blood pressure regulation, 14
   and high blood pressure, 20–23, 43
   tests for narrowing of, 45
Arteriosclerosis, 20, 146
Aspirin, 160
Asthma, 129
Atenolol, 128, 136
Atherosclerosis, 22, 146

B

Baroreceptors, 14
Benazepril, 130, 136
Bendroflumethiazide, 126, 136
Beta blockers, 128–129
   and alcohol, 114
   and anti-inflammatory drugs, 160
   and coronary artery disease, 147
   and hardened arteries, 146
   and heart failure, 147
   and high cholesterol, 148
   in hypertensive emergencies, 135
   in older adults, 145
   and pregnancy, 141
Betaxolol, 129
Bicycling, 66
Biofeedback, 123
Bisoprolol, 129, 136
Blood cell count, 44
Blood pressure
   chronic low, 19
   classification of, 17–18
   daily variation of, 16
   home monitoring, 153–157
   measuring, 15, 17, 38–40
   natural regulation of, 13–14
Body mass index, 52–54
Breathing exercises, 121–122
Bruit, 43
Bumetanide, 127
Bundle branch block, 129

Buproprion, 111

C
Caffeine, 114–116
Calcium
    and high blood pressure, 82
    sources of, 84
    supplements, 162
Calcium antagonists, 131–132, 145, 148
Calories
    activity guide, 68
    daily needs, 61
Captopril, 130, 136
Cardiovascular system, 12–13, 146–147
Carteolol, 129
Carvedilol, 129
Central-acting agents, 114, 133–134, 148
Children, 144
Chlorothiazide, 126
Chlorthalidone, 126, 136
Chinese food, 90
Cholesterol, 32, 44, 129, 148
Clonidine, 133
Coarctation, 34
Coenzyme Q-20, 162
Cold medicines, 161
Combination drugs, 135, 136, 164
Complications, 11, 20–26
Computed tomography (CT), 45
Condiments, 100–101
Cooking
    avoiding salt, 98–101
    reducing fat, 88
Coronary artery disease, 147
Cortisol, 118, 119
Counseling, 123
Creatinine, 44
Cross-country ski machines, 67

D
Deep breathing, 121–122
Diabetes, 32, 147–148
Diagnosing high blood pressure, 39–40
Diastolic pressure, 15–16

Diet pills, 161
Dietary Approaches to Stop Hypertension (DASH)
    menus and recipes, 167–181
    nutritional guidelines, 78–81
    study results, 77–78
Dieting. *See* Weight control
Digital monitors, 155
Diltiazem, 132, 136
Direct vasodilators, 134, 135
Directory of Prescription Drug Indigent Programs, 164
Diuretics, 126–128, 160
Doxazosin, 132
Drug interactions, 159–161
Drugs, illicit, 34–35, 43, 161
Drugs, injectable, 135
Dual metalloprotease inhibitors, 137

E
Eating well. *See* Nutrition
Eclampsia, 143
Edema, 24, 43
Electrocardiogram (ECG), 44
Electronic monitors, 155
Emergency warning signs, 151
Enalapril, 130, 136
Endothelin inhibitors, 137
Ephedrine, 162
Epinephrine, 14, 113, 118, 119
Esmolol hydrochloride, 135
Essential high blood pressure, 27–28
Estrogen, 140, 143
Ethacrynic acid, 127
Ethnic groups, 28, 145–146, 147
Evaluating high blood pressure, 40–45
Exercise. *See* Activity
Exercise machines, 66–67
Eyes, 26, 43

F
Family and friends, 165–166
Family history, 29, 41, 56
Felodipine, 132, 136
Fenoldopam, 135
Fibromuscular dysplasia, 34

Financial assistance, 164
Finger monitors, 155–156
Fish oil capsules, 162
Fitness plan, 69–75
Follow-up care, 164
Food additives, 95
Food labels
    nutrition labeling, 85–86, 98, 100
    sodium claims, 100
Fosinopril, 130
Furosemide, 127

G
Garlic, 162
Generic drugs, 161, 163
Genetic research, 138
Gestational hypertension, 141
Gingko biloba, 162
Gout, 127
Grapefruit juice, interactions with medications, 132, 161
Green tea, 162
Grocery shopping, 85–86, 87
Guanabenz, 133
Guanadrel, 133
Guanethidine, 133
Guanfacine, 133
Guided imagery, 123

H
Heart
    and blood pressure regulation, 14
    and high blood pressure, 23–24, 43
Heart failure, 24, 32, 43, 147
Hemorrhagic strokes, 25
Herbal supplements, 43, 162
High blood pressure (hypertension)
    in children, 144
    classification of, 17–18
    complications of, 11, 20–26
    emergency warning signs, 151
    essential vs. secondary, 27–28
    home monitoring, 153–157
    incidence of, 11, 139
    in older adults, 145
    resistant, 149–150
    symptoms of, 18, 20
Home monitoring, 153–157
    correct technique, 156–157
    equipment types, 154–156
Hormone replacement therapy, 143
Hydralazine, 134
Hydrochlorothiazide, 127, 136
Hypertensive emergency, 150–152
Hypotension, 19, 44
Hypothyroidism, 34

I
Ibuprofen, 160
Inactivity
    getting more active, 63–76
    health risks of, 30
Indapamide, 127
Insomnia, 116
Insulin, 52
Irbesartan, 130
Ischemic strokes, 24
Isolated systolic hypertension, 145
Isradipine, 132
Italian food, 90–91

J
Japanese food, 91
Jogging, 66

K
Ketoprofen, 160
Kidney disease
    and blood pressure medication, 148–149
    causing high blood pressure, 33
    tests for, 44
Kidneys
    and blood pressure regulation, 14, 25
    damage from high blood pressure, 25–26
    enlarged, 43

L
Labetalol, 129
Labetalol hydrochloride, 135

Laughter, 121
Left ventricular hypertrophy, 23
Licorice, 161, 162
Lifestyle changes
  activity, 63–76
  alcohol use, 112–114
  caffeine intake, 114–116
  eating well, 77–92
  importance of, 48–49
  smoking, 107–112
  sodium intake, 93–105
  stress, 117–124
  weight control, 51–61
Lisinopril, 130, 136
"Lite" salt, 105
Loop diuretics, 127, 148
Losartan potassium, 130, 136
Losing weight. See Weight control
Low blood pressure, 19, 44
Lupus, 134

M

Magnesium
  and arrhythmia, 146
  and high blood pressure, 82
  sources of, 84–85
  supplements, 162
Magnesium sulfate, 142
Magnetic resonance angiography (MRA), 45
Magnetic resonance imaging (MRI), 45
Mayo Clinic Health Oasis, 88, 137, 158
Measuring blood pressure, 15, 17, 38–40
Medications, 125–138
  Accupril (quinapril), 130
  acebutolol, 128
  Actron (ketoprofen), 160
  Adalat CC (nifedipine), 132
  Advil (ibuprofen), 160
  and alcohol use, 113–114
  Aldactazide, 136
  Aldactone (spironolactone), 127
  Aldomet (methyldopa), 134
  Alka-Seltzer, 100
  allergy medicines, 161

Medications — cont'd
  Altace (ramipril), 130
  amiloride, 127, 136
  amlodipine, 132, 136
  Apresoline (hydralazine), 134
  Aquatensen (methyclothiazide), 127
  aspirin, 160
  atenolol, 128, 136
  Avapro (irbesartan), 130
  benazepril, 130, 136
  bendroflumethiazide, 126, 136
  betaxolol, 129
  bisoprolol, 129, 136
  Blocadren (timolol), 129
  Bromo Seltzer, 100
  bulk purchases, 163–164
  bumetanide, 127
  Bumex (bumetanide), 127
  buproprion, 111
  Calan SR (verapamil), 132
  Capoten (captopril), 130
  Capozide, 136
  captopril, 130, 136
  Cardene SR (nicardipine), 132
  Cardizem CD (diltiazem), 132
  Cardizem SR (diltiazem), 132
  Cardura (doxazosin), 132
  carteolol, 129
  Cartrol (carteolol), 129
  carvedilol, 129
  Catapres (clonidine), 133
  causing high blood pressure, 34, 43
  chlorothiazide, 126
  chlorthalidone, 126, 136
  classes of, 126
  clonidine, 133
  cold medicines, 161
  combination drugs, 135, 136, 164
  Coreg (carvedilol), 129
  Corgard (nadolol), 129
  Corzide, 136
  Covera HS (verapamil), 132
  Cozaar (losartan potassium), 130
  Demadex (torsemide), 127
  diet pills, 161

Medications — cont'd
  Dilacor XR (diltiazem), 132
  diltiazem, 132, 136
  Diovan HCT, 136
  Diovan (valsartan), 130
  Diulo (metolazone), 127
  Diuril (chlorothiazide), 126
  doxazosin, 132
  drug interactions, 159–161
  Dyazide, 136
  DynaCirc (isradipine), 132
  DynaCirc CR (isradipine), 132
  Dyrenium (triamterene), 127
  Edecrin (ethacrynic acid), 127
  enalapril, 130, 136
  Enduron (methyclothiazide), 127
  Esidrix (hydrochlorothiazide), 127
  esmolol hydrochloride, 135
  ethacrynic acid, 127
  felodipine, 132, 136
  fenoldopam, 135
  financial assistance, 164
  fosinopril, 130
  furosemide, 127
  generic, 161, 163
  grapefruit juice interactions, 161
  guanabenz, 133
  guanadrel, 133
  guanethidine, 133
  guanfacine, 133
  hydralazine, 134
  hydrochlorothiazide, 127, 136
  Hydrodiuril (hydrochloroth-
    iazide), 127
  Hygroton (chlorthalidone), 126
  Hylorel (guanadrel), 133
  Hytrin (terazosin), 132
  Hyzaar, 136
  ibuprofen, 160
  indapamide, 127
  Inderal (propranolol), 129
  Inderal LA (propranolol), 129
  Inderide LA, 136
  injectable drugs, 135
  irbesartan, 130
  Ismelin (guanethidine), 133

Medications — cont'd
  Isoptin SR (verapamil), 132
  isradipine, 132
  Kerlone (betaxolol), 129
  ketoprofen, 160
  labetalol, 129
  labetalol hydrochloride, 135
  Lasix (furosemide), 127
  Levatol (penbutolol), 129
  Lexxel, 136
  lisinopril, 130, 136
  Loniten (minoxidil), 134
  Lopressor HCT, 136
  Lopressor (metoprolol), 129
  losartan potassium, 130, 136
  Lotensin (benazepril), 130
  Lotensin HCT, 136
  Lotrel, 136
  Lozol (indapamide), 127
  magnesium sulfate, 142
  Mavik (trandolapril), 130
  Maxzide, 136
  methyclothiazide, 127
  methyldopa, 133, 134, 141
  metolazone, 127
  metoprolol, 129, 136
  Microzide (hydrochlorothiazide),
    127
  Midamor (amiloride), 127
  Minipress (prazosin), 132
  minoxidil, 134
  Moduretic, 136
  moexipril, 130
  Monopril (fosinopril), 130
  Motrin-IB (ibuprofen), 160
  Mykrox (metolazone), 127
  nadolol, 129, 136
  Naprosyn (naproxen sodium), 160
  Naturetin (bendroflumethiazide),
    126
  nicardipine, 132
  nicardipine hydrochloride, 135
  nifedipine, 132
  nitroglycerin, 135
  Normodyne (labetalol), 129
  Norvasc (amlodipine), 132

Medications — cont'd
  Oretic (hydrochlorothiazide), 127
  Orudis-KT (ketoprofen), 160
  penbutolol, 129
  phentolamine, 135
  pindolol, 129
  Plendil (felodipine), 132
  prazosin, 132
  Prinivil (lisinopril), 130
  Prinzide, 136
  Procardia XL (nifedipine), 132
  propranolol, 129, 136
  quinapril, 130
  ramipril, 130
  research, 137–138
  reserpine, 134
  Sectral (acebutolol), 128
  Serpasil (reserpine), 134
  side effects, 127–134
  sodium nitroprusside, 135
  spironolactone, 127, 136
  splitting pills, 163
  Tarka, 136
  Teczem, 136
  Tenex (guanfacine), 133
  Tenoretic, 136
  Tenormin (atenolol), 128
  terazosin, 132
  Thalitone (chlorthalidone), 126
  Tiazac (diltiazem), 132
  timolol, 129
  tips, 158–159
  Toprol XL (metoprolol), 129
  torsemide, 127
  Trandate (labetalol), 129
  trandolapril, 130, 136
  triamterene, 127, 136
  types, 126
  Univasc (moexipril), 130
  valsartan, 130, 136
  Vaseretic, 136
  Vasotec (enalapril), 130
  verapamil, 132, 136
  Verelan (verapamil), 132
  Visken (pindolol), 129
  Wytensin (guanabenz), 133

Medications — cont'd
  Zaroxolyn (metolazone), 127
  Zebeta (bisoprolol), 129
  Zestoretic, 136
  Zestril (lisinopril), 130
  Ziac, 136
  Zyban (buprorion), 111
Meditation, 123
Menus, 167–174
Mercury-column monitors, 154
Methyclothiazide, 127
Methyldopa, 133, 134, 141
Metolazone, 127
Metoprolol, 129, 136
Mexican food, 91
Minoxidil, 134
Moexipril, 130
Monitoring equipment, 154–156
Monosodium glutamate (MSG), 90, 100
Muscle tension exercises, 122–123

N

Nadolol, 129, 136
Natriuretic peptide clearance inhibitors, 137
Nicardipine, 132
Nicardipine hydrochloride, 135
Nicotine, 108
Nicotine replacements, 111
Nifedipine, 132
Nitroglycerin, 135
Norepinephrine, 128
Nuclear scanning, 45
Nutrition
  calcium sources, 84
  cooking techniques, 88
  DASH guidelines, 78–81
  DASH menus and recipes, 167–181
  food labels, 85–86
  potassium sources, 82–83
  restaurant meals, 89–91
  shopping tips, 85, 87
  sodium recommendations, 96–97, 98, 100–105
Nutritional supplements, 43, 162

O

Obesity
    definition of, 52–53
    risks of, 29–30
Omega-3 fatty acids, 80–81, 162
Oral contraceptives, 140
Organ damage, signs of, 43

P

Penbutolol, 129
Perceived Exertion Scale, 65
Phentolamine, 135
Physical activity. *See* Activity
Pindolol, 129
Positive thinking, 121
Postural hypotension, 19, 44
Potassium
    and arrhythmia, 146
    blood chemistry tests, 44
    potassium-sparing diuretics, 127–128
    and sodium regulation, 31
    sources of, 82–83
    supplements, 162
Potassium chloride, 105
Potassium-sparing diuretics, 105, 127
Prazosin, 132
Preeclampsia, 34, 142–143
Pregnancy, 34, 130, 131, 140–143
Propranolol, 129, 136
Pseudohypertension, 39

Q

Quitting smoking, 109–112
Quinapril, 130

R

Race. *See* Ethnic groups
Ramipril, 130
Recipes, 175–181
Relaxation, 121–123, 124
Renin inhibitors, 137
Research, medications, 137–138
Reserpine, 134
Resistant high blood pressure, 149–150
Restaurant meals, 89–91
Risk factors, 28–33, 47
Risk groups, 46–48
Rowing machines, 67

S

Salt. *See* Sodium
Salt substitutes, 105
Seasonings, 99, 100, 104–105
Secondary high blood pressure, 33–35, 42
Side effects of medications, 127–134
Sleep, 120
Sleep apnea, 32, 150
Smoking, 107–112
Social relationships, 121, 165–166
Sodium
    blood chemistry tests, 44
    controversial studies, 97
    dietary recommendations, 96–97, 98, 100–105
    food additives, 95
    food labels, 98, 100
    and high blood pressure, 31
Sodium nitroprusside, 135
Sodium sensitivity, 31, 94, 96
Soy sauce, 91
Sphygmomanometer, 15, 38
Spironolactone, 127, 136
Splitting pills, 163
Spring-gauge monitors, 154–155
Stair-climber machines, 67
Stationary bicycles, 67
Strengthening exercises, 73–74
Stress, 117–124
    and blood pressure, 32, 117, 119
    body's response to, 118–119
    coping with, 119–124
    and overall health, 120
Stretching, 70–72, 123
Stroke, 24–25
Swelling, 24, 43
Swimming, 66
Symptoms, 18, 20
Systolic pressure, 15

T

Terazosin, 132
Tests, 44–45
Thiazides, 126–127, 146, 148
Thyroid disease, 33–34
Timolol, 129
Tobacco use, 31, 107–112
Torsemide, 127
Toxemia. *See* Preeclampsia
Trandolapril, 130, 136
Treadmills, 67
Treatment guidelines, 46–48
    follow-up care, 164
Triamterene, 127, 136
"Type A" personality, 117

U

Ultrasonography, 45
Urinalysis, 44

V

Valsartan, 130, 136
Vasopressin antagonists, 138
Verapamil, 132, 136
Visualization, 123
Vitamin C, 162

W

Walking, 65–66
Weight control, 51–62
    activity guide, 68
    body mass index, 52–53
    calorie needs, 61
    commercial programs, 59
    healthy weight, 55–56
    steps for success, 58–61
Weight lifting, 74
"White-coat" hypertension, 41, 150, 154
Wrist monitors, 155–156

Y

Yohimbine, 162